A New Body

IN ONE DAY

A Guide to Same-Day
Cosmetic Surgery Procedures

DISCARD

by

Robert A. Yoho, M.D.
and Judy Brandy-Yoho, R.N.

with Terri Mandell

A NEW BODY IN ONE DAY:
A Guide to Same-Day
Cosmetic Surgery Procedures

by Robert A. Yoho, M.D., and Judy Brandy-Yoho, R.N.,
with Terri Mandell

Edited by Terri Mandell
Copy edited by Vivian Margolin
Text design by Terri Mandell, Jim Mandell,
and Sue Kientz
Front and back cover design by Gregg Heard
Back cover photography by Michael Jacobs

First Edition: March 1997
Second Printing: September 1998

ISBN 0-9659541-0-2
Library of Congress Catalog #96-086488

Published by
Inverness Press
675 S. Arroyo Parkway, Suite 100
Pasadena, CA 91105
tel: (626) 585-0800 fax: (626) 585-8887

With Gratitude . . .

This book is dedicated to our first child, Hannah Elizabeth Yoho.

We would like to thank the people who have helped us with the development of our cosmetic surgery practice, and who have helped us make this book possible. Terri Mandell was the creative force that supported us throughout the project. Greg Heard's cover artwork is absolutely first rate.

Dr. Mani Nambiar wrote and rewrote the chapters on breast reconstruction, nose surgery, and face lifts. Riad Roomi, M.D., a plastic surgeon from London, had particularly incisive comments about cellulite. Alan Chun, M.D., a highly skilled maxilofacial surgeon, wrote the chin improvement section, and Alan Ho a Shoo rewrote some of the laser information to reflect the latest technologies.

At Image Realm, our printer James Gonzales and his staff are truly artists, with an outstanding eye for detail. The inside color pages were a labor of dedication for Adam Gonzalez, whose expertise and patience are the stuff all should seek to achieve.

I want to express my appreciation to my physician mentors, in alphabetical order and a partial listing. Bill Cook is one of the great names in our field and generous with his time. Gary Fenno was a mentor to many of us. Jim Fulton is a unique friend, mentor, and medical innovator. When I get discouraged, I visit him for a course or a day, and I get a recharge that lasts for months. Modern liposuctionists everywhere owe a debt to Jeff Klein, for innovations in anesthetic technique and cannula design. He allowed me to observe him during my first year in practice. Pat Lillis has been extraordinarily kind to me throughout my career, his strongest influence being on my technique, and I feel he is much less recognized nationally than he deserves. Barry Miller's experience extends from nearly the beginning of our field, and he allowed me into his Honolulu office early on. Michael Rabkin kindly helped me learn some of his unique laser bleharoplasty techniques. Dow Stough gave me my start in hair transplantation. He combines an academic career with an extremely busy private practice; I don't know how he does it.

Our office staff and patients gave us suggestions, moral support, and enormous enthusiasm. Thanks to my surgical assistant, Dr. Kevin Chiasson, who also helped provide the newest photos. Chic Holtkamp, Lenore Kaddish, Dr. L.R. Friedman, Shiela Heckman, Betty Holst, Christine Farmer, Gary Grasso, Joyce Meadows, Miriam Dexter, Jeff Baird, and my father Alan Yoho, M.D., all reviewed the text and offered useful suggestions. Becky Craig, Sue Kientz, and Vivian Margolin all contributed to the editing and proofreading of the text, and corrected deficiencies in my writing skills. Many other people gave suggestions, including many of our patients. For their help and encouragement we are very appreciative.

Author's Introduction

Much of what's written about cosmetic surgery in newspapers and magazines, and even in some medical journals, is half-truth, myth, or advertising. The media has distorted public perception with overly negative or sensationalized stories, and medical specialty organizations contribute to the mayhem by promoting warring viewpoints to establish their own market share. The misinformation is further compounded by the rapid pace of technological change. As soon as we begin to understand one procedure, new ones pop up, and the confusion begins anew. Many of today's finest techniques didn't even exist five years ago. And five years from now, these may be ancient history.

On top of that, a patient's psychological perspective is often ignored, and this, in many ways, is the most important aspect of the whole process. That's why I've chosen to open the book with a chapter called "The Psychology of Cosmetic Surgery." Motivation, media influence, culture, expectations, family pressures, and other factors have an enormous influence on one's perceptions and decisions.

On the physical side, the safety of cosmetic surgery is better than it's ever been, thanks to recent innovations in anesthesia and other techniques. A new kind of numbing medicine known as "tumescent anesthesia" was introduced only a few years ago and is now becoming a new standard. General anesthesia, which involves heavier drugs, intensive (and expensive) medical supervision, and sometimes a more difficult recovery, is now often unnecessary. With the new local anesthesia, side effects such as nausea, drugged feelings, and a sense of losing control can usually be avoided. But the best news is that your surgery can now be done in an outpatient surgical center, and you can go home only a few hours later with a new body. *In one day.*

Having one of these procedures performed under local anesthetic also gives you the option of observing what's going on in the room. It's like watching a chef in the kitchen or an artist in the studio while he works — on you. You are awake and aware, but feeling little or no discomfort. You may also be able to speak with the doctor and the assistants, and that kind of communication can actually make it a very positive experience.

In this book you'll read detailed descriptions of what to expect from a variety of procedures, including specifics on how each procedure is done, what drugs are used, how you'll feel, and what the recovery will be like. You must be aware, however, that *no surgery is ever totally risk-free.* If you are planning to have cosmetic surgery, you *must* read chapter 16 on complications. This is a blunt and realistic assessment of the potential for problems, if any, after surgery. If you don't fully understand this information, you should go no further.

I've also included a chapter on choosing a cosmetic surgeon, with specific, honest information you won't find anywhere else. Choosing a physician can be a stressful experience because, frankly, doctors can be intimidating. They speak a different language, and they seem to live in a different world. They know things that most people don't know, and sometimes they wield a lot of power. Some of them are wealthy. Or famous. Many don't have enough experience in the exact surgery you're inquiring about, and some won't be able to take the time to answer all your questions. So how can you tell which doctors are skilled, experienced, and caring, and which are not? I'll give you some guidelines that can be useful for the rest of your life, beyond your cosmetic surgery experience.

Finally, it's important that you know that I've been a cosmetic surgery patient myself. In 1992 I had abdominal liposuction, and in 1995 I had a second liposuction to "fine tune" my result. I've also had a deep facial acid peel to get rid of some acne scars. This was done in the days before laser was used, when the procedure was called a "chemical peel." Recoveries from this were pretty brutal and less predictable than with today's technology. With the laser, it's a breeze by comparison.

I believe I have a unique perspective which helps me to see my patients' points of view. I'm aware of what they're feeling. I understand their apprehensions, their physical responses, and their expectations. I'm writing from the empathetic yet realistic viewpoint of a physician, with the added understanding of someone who has also been a patient.

This is a complicated field. There's been an explosion of interest, and at the same time, continuous little revolutions in the technology. My hope is that you will find enough clarity here to sort out the facts. As a cosmetic physician, my goal is to help you look and feel your best. But I also want to do *my* best to make sure you've done your homework.

For your continuing medical education,

Robert Yoho, M. D.

Robert A. Yoho, M.D.

Books Don't Do Surgery — Doctors Do

A Disclaimer

ଡ଼ *Rely on your doctor, not this book, for your final decisions about your surgery and care!*

I've tried to make this book as complete and accurate as possible, hoping to give enough general information to help you feel more knowledgeable about cosmetic surgery. But it's possible that between the day my words were written and the day you pulled this book from the bookstore shelf, medical advances may have changed some of these techniques. And although I have faith in the results these procedures can produce in good hands, any technique can be performed poorly. Even with the best of medical care, some patients just don't get the results they expect.

You'll see that I have very strong opinions about which techniques I prefer. Given expert care, even the dated techniques which I *don't* like — tummy tucks, trans-cutaneous blepharoplasty, major scalp surgery for hair loss, and phenol facial peels — have the potential for good and even excellent results for some patients.

These are still actively performed and advocated by many well-meaning physicians (but keep in mind there is a bigger range of "proper" technique for the art of cosmetic surgery than for other medical areas, such as heart disease). Also, some of the procedures which I *do* like — such as the Coleman facial fat injection — haven't been widely used yet, but I believe that they will be in the near future.

I respect the opinions of other doctors. The chapters on face lifts, nose reconstruction, and breast reconstruction were contributed by my associate, Dr. Mani Nambiar, and you will notice that he and I disagree on some minor points.

There are many other books in the marketplace which address cosmetic surgery, but my research has revealed that most of them are not written by physicians, and I believe that much of the information they contain is questionable. While doctors have a vested interest (we want to help you with your problems *and* get paid for it), we've also spent decades on our training and are held to a high standard by our medical licenses and personal ethics. So gather your information from multiple sources, read all the books you want, but ultimately, find a physician who makes you feel comfortable, and allow that person, and *only* that person, to help you finalize your cosmetic surgery decisions.

Contents

The Psychology of Cosmetic Surgery

  Cosmetic surgery patients often have very complex motivations, reactions, and psychology. But most of them have positive outcomes — in other words, their self-esteem and confidence are enhanced at a reasonable price in dollars and inconvenience.

  Despite this, some very negative books and articles have been written about this subject. I'm not from that universe — I'm optimistic about our ability to generate positive changes with our work.

  The recovery may be difficult psychologically for a minority of patients (of course, with our modern techniques, serious complications are less frequent than ever before).

  Physicians should provide emotional support along with cosmetic surgery. It's important for a doctor to spend enough time with each patient and to be truly caring.

  Our final goal is to have the physical improvement boost the patient's self esteem.

While most medical specialties address the physical body, cosmetic surgery is unique in the way it brings together elements of the physical and the psychological. It is, after all, the ultimate *elective* surgery, because a patient clearly chooses it voluntarily. And the patient's motivation — to look and feel better — is directly connected to his or her sense of self-worth. That's why I've chosen to put this chapter at the beginning of the book. Because physicians and patients both need to consider motivation, expectations and other psychological influences before making a cosmetic surgery commitment.

The true bottom line when making your decision about cosmetic surgery is simple — how much does the "flawed" area of your body bother you? If heavy thighs, small breasts or a receding hairline make you unhappy, then what else do you need to know? You're a free-thinking adult with decision-making power. You care about yourself. You want to improve the way you look and the way you feel. It's that simple. Or is it?

You'd be surprised at what happens when you scratch the surface of a simple thought like, "I'd like to look more attractive." Underneath that thought, all kinds of subconscious messages — cultural, sexual, social and physical — are screaming for attention. How do you sort them out so that each can be clearly heard?

Motivations For Cosmetic Surgery

The great news about motivation is that the vast majority of patients are not having cosmetic surgery to please someone else. They're doing it strictly for themselves, and that's a wonderful, healthy reason. The best reason.

We are motivated toward change by many things — a divorce, the need to accelerate in our careers, the expectations of spouses, family, or friends, cultural messages, and the influence of the media. These can all contribute to the decision to surgically change our appearance. But the best candidates for cosmetic surgery are those who take all that into consideration, and ultimately choose it for their own personal satisfaction. This is particularly true for patients who have medical conditions which cause deformities of the face or body. Their motivation is especially pure.

They want to survive emotionally in a world where they will most likely be shunned because of physical attributes over which they have no control.

I also see many patients who are recovering from a terrible life trauma, like the death of a spouse or abandonment by a spouse. In these cases, a change in physical appearance can provide a desperately-needed boost for self esteem. Some patients come from backgrounds of verbal or even physical abuse, and find that they've duplicated a childhood situation in their adult relationships by choosing partners who reaffirm their sense of unworthiness. One young woman's boyfriend constantly told her that she looked too old and wrinkled for him. Another woman's husband teased her mercilessly about her thighs. Many have had spouses who've left them for younger lovers, and others are struggling to make it up a corporate ladder where they're in direct competition with younger executives. Finally, many patients — and most people who may never become patients — are simply locked into the belief that younger is better. Thinner is better. Large breasts are better. More hair is better.

Our goal as physicians, when we change our patients' bodies, is to enable them to use their personal power more effectively. A larger pair of breasts does not guarantee that a woman will attract the man of her dreams. A new head of hair does not guarantee that a man will be the center of attention at a party. But the combination of better looks (which lead to a better self image), and a positive response from other people, can produce more personal confidence and effectiveness.

Depression and Cosmetic Surgery

A marketing consultant I know designed a brochure for a psychologist named Dr. Jefferies, who was building a unique counseling practice in Beverly Hills working exclusively with women who'd had cosmetic surgery. The headline on Dr. Jefferies' brochure read, "Now That I'm Beautiful, Why Do I Still Feel So Sad?"

That was in 1989, when many of the procedures discussed in this book were performed less frequently, and cosmetic surgery was often viewed as an option for only the very rich or the very vain. The women who came to Dr. Jefferies had one thing in common. They'd approached their cosmetic surgeries at the time when annihilating events like being dumped by their husbands for younger women, led them to take what in those days was considered a desperate measure. Many of the women in failing marriages were convinced that slimming their bodies with liposuction or erasing some of their wrinkles would make things better. They were half right. It did make their bodies better. But it didn't always keep their husbands at home. It didn't necessarily alleviate their depression.

The modern cosmetic surgeon has the chance during the initial consultation to recognize and treat these patients. He ideally looks at the patient's psyche along with the physique, and will recognize depression when present. Depression is a real medical condition. There can be physical problems lasting months to years which include sadness, sleep disturbance, difficulty feeling pleasure, and sometimes other signs such as stomach problems or diarrhea. Fully 20 percent of the population will experience depression at some time in their lives. In our practice, if appropriate and if the patient wishes, we treat these patients with modern antidepressants like Prozac® and its relatives. The cosmetic procedure and the medication can be used together, and when this happens, the transformations can often be profound. Given the right candidates (and they're common), the medications work well in many cases and even miraculously in some. People who weren't very functional find their lives turned around, and people who were very functional often become more so. Between the medication and the body improvement, a "moth" may change into a "butterfly" in just a few weeks, although in more severe cases of depression, surgery might not be recommended until the depression is treated.

Stresses and Emotional Factors During the Immediate Recovery

It's hard to completely prepare our patients for their experiences, because each individual's reaction is unique. Most people sail through the recovery without incident, and although pain isn't usually a big deal, in a minority of cases, it can be significant. For example, with our liposuction patients, 95 percent need only Tylenol® the night after the surgery. For the other five percent, recovery involves taking heavier medications for a couple of days. Patients who have used heavy doses of prescription pain killers in the past may experience more pain. And people who have had major physical experiences such as childbirth often find cosmetic surgery discomfort a breeze. And recovery — as with any stress — is easier for those individuals in good overall physical and emotional health.

Our patients are warned to expect a brief depression a week to a month after the surgery, because body image distortion during the recovery period can be particularly difficult. This is a temporary stress rather than a full-blown depression needing medication. With facial fat transplants, for example, there is generally little physical pain, but the swelling (at its worst the first two to three weeks) can be disheartening until the new face appears. Use of a hyperbaric chamber can shorten this difficult period (please see chapter 17 on the hyperbaric chamber).

Depression can also occur if there are complications, when the whole process demands more time and energy than patients have budgeted for emotionally (see chapter 16 on complications). For example, an infection, facial nerve injury or eyelid problem, though rare, can happen occasionally even with the best of care. In these cases, a recovery that should have taken weeks can drag out for months, and possibly longer.

For some people — five to ten percent or less, depending on the procedure — cosmetic surgery recovery is emotionally demanding. Your physician should make sure you are prepared for the possibility of depression. What you should *not* expect from your physician is psychoanalysis, a warning about every psychological reaction before it happens, or even necessarily antidepressant medications. You should expect compassion, professionalism, emotional support and thorough, sensitive follow-up to help you deal with your reactions, whatever they may be.

Can Changing Your Body Change Your Life?

When people ask me, "Should I have this done?" I ask them, "How bad does it make you feel, and how much better would you feel if it were changed?"

The body and the mind work together, and our hope is that helping the body will help the mind. For example, some of our liposuction patients go back to the gym with their new bodies and for the first time are able to work out without shame. Their workouts burn calories, and instead of continuing to spiral down into depression and inaction, they begin to lose weight and feel better. After a laser peel, a more youthful face can generate new confidence and improve spirits. Some people are able to make all kinds of lifestyle changes, such as getting married or divorced, finding a new boyfriend, or taking a major career risk. After a hair transplant, men may feel better on their jobs and feel more attractive to the opposite sex. The combination of improved appearance, new confidence, and the reactions of other people can contribute to positive changes in a cosmetic surgery patient's life.

But there's another side to the story. Some patients, after surgery, will be less able to deal with the possibility of changes in their lives. For example, if after liposuction you continue lifelong bad eating habits, and return to fat-laden foods, sugary snacks and no exercise, you will gain weight. On the emotional side, a new body image has the potential to force you to face difficult issues, such as changes in sexual relationships or less-than-supportive responses from friends and family. People may treat you differently after the surgery, and there is the occasional family member or friend who will resent you for looking and feeling better. A surgeon's *hope* is that the improvements will contribute to a better emotional life for the patient. The surgeon's *responsibility* is to counsel and advise patients on how to adopt the healthiest possible lifestyle.

Men and Cosmetic Surgery

Cosmetic surgery, once considered the exclusive domain of women, is now requested more and more by men. While in 1980, only about a tenth of all cosmetic procedures were performed on men, this number has now increased to 25 percent or more.

Hair transplants are the most common procedure sought by men, and results have become more natural-looking over the past five years. Something happens at a very basic level when it comes to men and their hair. Some men who are balding feel that they're losing touch with a powerful prime directive, as if their strength and purpose are being compromised. Imagine a male lion without a mane. Or a male peacock without his beautiful colors. There are some profound masculine insights in the story of Samson and Delilah. It may have to do with sexual drives or fears about aging, but whatever the underlying psychology, it's a powerful force for our male patients.

The Ambivalence Factor: Fear and Guilt

Dr. Kate Altork, a psychotherapist who specializes in working with cosmetic surgery patients, gave a talk at the January 1996 meeting of the American Academy of Cosmetic Surgeons (AACS). She beautifully addressed some of the emotional issues that affect the decision-making process. I have paraphrased her ideas in this section, while including some of my own.

Seldom do people unconditionally love their appearance. But the prospect of changing it brings feelings of guilt and fear. The fear is easy to identify. The guilt is a little harder. To understand each one clearly, let's look at them one at a time.

The fear begins during the initial consultation. Patients often sit in the waiting room in a state of hyper-vigilance, eyeing every patient who comes through the door, watching staff members suspiciously, and listening acutely to every sound. Their fear is not hard to understand. As a patient, you're considering having a total stranger permanently alter your face or body. There are dozens of questions going through your mind. What if something goes terribly wrong? What if there's a mistake, and you're disfigured for life? Is it going to hurt? What if the horror stories in the media are true?

The next step is meeting the doctor face-to-face. In the consultation room, you will have to reveal one of the most vulnerable parts of yourself to this intimidating stranger. The sagging stomach you've tried to hide with loose clothing for years is now going to be inspected closely by someone you don't even know. Or he's going to scrutinize your wrinkles, or study the bags under your eyes, and make comments about how these things can be "fixed." You feel as though you're being judged. If the doctor has an inadequate understanding of patients' feelings, if he lacks compassion, if he lacks the ability to make you feel emotionally safe, the consultation has the potential to feel humiliating.

The Seven Guilt Messages

Guilt can be stimulated by many factors. Why do we humans feel guilty about loving ourselves? Some of the answers can be plainly seen when we look at the cultural, religious, social, sexual and media influences on our lives. Here's a breakdown of messages that prompt us to feel guilty for altering our physical appearance:

1. *We should accept what nature gave us*

    Many of us were taught that we should accept ourselves just as nature made us. We were also taught, rightly so, that what's inside a person is more important than what's on the outside. In early childhood we learned clichés such as, "You can't judge a book by it's cover," and "Beauty's only skin deep."

2. *Vanity is bad*

    Some believe that vanity is a sin, which plays beautifully into the fear, "Will I be punished for my vanity by a disastrous result from the surgery?"

3. *It's an extravagant use of money*

    How can you spend thousands of dollars on cosmetic surgery when you really need a new roof on the house? What kind of person would spend that kind of money on himself when there are children starving?

4. *Cosmetic surgery is dishonest*

    If we really believe that beauty's only skin deep, then we're dishonest if we surgically alter our appearance. Our new attractiveness will be false.

5. Cosmetic surgery is not politically correct

Are you buying the media myth about how you should look? Many female baby boomers believed in the "natural look" during the 1970s. They stopped wearing make up, and many stopped shaving their legs and underarms. Now that they're in their 40s and 50s, are they compromising their ethics? Shouldn't we be proud of the age, experience and wisdom that shows in our faces?

6. What will people think?

We want to be taken seriously by our peers. We want to be seen as deep, intelligent people. So how can we justify something as "shallow" as having our breasts enlarged? Public opinion seems to hold the view that cosmetic surgery is for insecure high-society types, desperate women, bimbos or people who are obsessively afraid of aging. Who wants to be one of "them?"

7. The media monster

The media constantly reminds us that cosmetic surgery is for the rich and famous, not for regular folks like us. We see it in the gossip pages. We see it in the advertising of cosmetic surgeons. In most of the hype, we see pictures of 23-year-old female fashion models with perfect bodies. We don't see ourselves in these images. We see people we can't relate to, so we're sold an idea that says, "Cosmetic surgery is for the young, beautiful, famous or rich." Seldom do the ads show middle aged men and women, adolescents with disfigurements, or average looking people with obvious flaws.

These ads make us feel guilty twice. The first pang of guilt is because we feel as if we've let ourselves get fat and bald and didn't work hard enough to maintain our youthful appearance. The second pang comes when we start thinking about having cosmetic surgery, and the whole cycle begins all over again with "we should accept what nature gave us."

Deciding to undergo cosmetic surgery is not an easy process. The odds can seem stacked against you when you consider all the elements described in this chapter. The average cosmetic surgery patient begins thinking about having surgery four years before making inquiries, and then has two to three consultations with different doctors before deciding. I think this makes good sense.

Look in the mirror and listen to your feelings. How much better would you feel if you could streamline your shape, grow new hair, enhance your breasts or lose those facial jowls? Would it build your confidence? Would you function more effectively in the world if you could feel *good* about the way you look? And if so, how realistic are your expectations? If you're over 40, ask yourself, "Do I want to look like a young fashion model, or do I want to look the best I can *for my age?*" If you feel certain that cosmetic surgery will help you feel better, and if you're willing to take good care of yourself physically and emotionally once you've made the change, then congratulations! You've made a decision based on self-respect and wisdom.

A new body by itself can't guarantee career success, an improved social life or a more stable marriage. It won't solve your everyday problems. But it's one part of a process of growth, change and improvement to the whole self that we engage in throughout our lives.

Choosing Your Cosmetic Surgeon 2

There's an old expression which says, "The best way to judge a man is to meet his dog." If the man in question happens to be a physician to whom you're entrusting your body, then this axiom would apply to his staff, his patients, his family, and anyone else who reflects his personality. If the people around him are unhappy or unhealthy, if they appear to be untrustworthy, cold or rude, then this should give you a good indication of what the doctor is like. Another consideration is whether the doctor and his staff seem truly interested in their jobs. A doctor who loves what he's doing can help you feel more confident about your decision.

There are many factors to consider when choosing a physician of any kind, but your own emotional response is the most critical index of how safe you're going to feel with this person. Because there are so many factors to consider, and because choosing the right doctor is such an important part of the surgical process, I've broken this chapter down into sections covering the most important elements.

Be Procedure Specific

Each doctor's practice has a personality, and each doctor excels at something specific. Find out which procedure(s) the doctor performs most often, and if it's the one you're interested in, then pursue it. Before you get to the point where you actually go to the office for a consultation, you can narrow your choices down considerably in one easy step: ask questions that are "procedure specific."

Most physicians have a few procedures in which they are the most experienced. A good place to start is with a doctor who specializes full-time in cosmetic surgery (some do ordinary injury and surgical care as well).

Ask, for example, "How many liposuctions have you done?" You might want to take it one step further and ask, "How many liposuctions have you done on someone my age, with my coloring?" If a cosmetic surgeon has done a thousand, but you're looking for a facial laser peel and he's only done 50, then he may not be right for you. Your best bet is to find an ultra-specialist. Some of these procedures (noses and liposuction in particular) have learning curves up to 1,000 procedures long. *Experience is almost everything.*

On a personal note, recently I needed to have hernia repair surgery. I decided to have it done through a flexible scope (endoscopic hernia repair), and I consulted three physicians, all of whom had performed several thousand cases. I chose the one who inspired the greatest measure of confidence. I suggest you follow this model, and choose someone who's had extensive experience in the *exact* procedure you want, and who you *feel* is right for you.

Look at the Right Kind of Before-and-After Photos

A cosmetic surgeon should *always* let you see before-and-after photos of his patients. If he says he doesn't have any, for whatever reason, look elsewhere.

When you're looking at photos, don't just settle for a random handful of shots. You need to look at dozens — maybe even hundreds — to get a good sense of the doctor's work. Ask to see very specific types of photos, for example, shots of people who've had the *exact* procedure you're planning to have, and who have bodies similar to yours (skin condition, skin color, body weight, shape, and age).

Speak with Other Patients

First, ask the doctor directly what percentage of his patients are referred to him *by other patients*. The best practices get the majority of their patients by referral. If most of the patients come in response to advertising alone, you may want to think twice. Ask the doctor or the staff if they'll give you the phone numbers of some other patients who've had the same procedure you're inquiring about, including some operated on in the past month. A percentage of these patients should be agreeable to providing support to newcomers. If the doctor says he cannot let you talk to his patients, this is a bad sign. There are no better information sources on earth than people who've had the same surgery.

Another way to learn about the doctor's expertise is to "socialize" in his waiting room. Show up 30 minutes early for your consultation, and spend some time questioning patients in the waiting room. You'll find that most cosmetic surgery patients are very willing to talk about what they've had done. If you see a woman with a bandaged face, ask her how she feels and what kind of procedure she had. If you tell her that you're considering the same thing, she'll probably be happy to share her impressions with you. Ask her what she thinks of the doctor and the staff. Ask her how available they were for follow-up and how responsive they were *after* the procedure. The staff should be more than happy to let you speak with other patients.

The Scoop on Specialty Boards

Cosmetic surgery techniques change rapidly, and the technology is always new. Even someone who was board certified as recently as five years ago may not be up to speed on the narrow specialty field of an individual procedure. Certain specialty boards promote themselves as being somehow superior to others, and some claim that no other physicians but those in their group should be doing surgery at all. But this is wrong. Dermatologists, plastic surgeons, ophthalmologists, ear-nose-throat specialists and others have *all* contributed to the development of modern cosmetic surgery. Competent physicians can be found in each group.

If I had to generalize about specialties, the following are my recommendations. But bear in mind that modern training cuts across specialty lines, and is as recent as yesterday.

Ear-nose-throat specialists who've had an extra year of cosmetic surgery training might be able to do the best "nose jobs." They can do a great job with the functional breathing apparatus as well as make you look better.

Plastic surgeons also often do a great job with noses, and generally have years of training for breast reconstructions of all kinds. Most liposuction has been done in recent years by dermatologists, but now plastic surgeons have, in many cases, adopted the new "tumescent" anesthesia, which was developed originally by Drs. Klein and Lillis (both dermatologists). For laser work, dermatologists generally have the most experience, but many other specialty fields are getting involved. Eyelid surgery (blepharoplasty) is performed by dermatologists, plastic surgeons, and also by ophthalmologists specially trained in a field called "oculo-plastics." Hair transplantation physicians come from many specialties.

I can't emphasize strongly enough how important it is for a doctor to be up to date on new procedures, techniques, drugs and other vital information. Things change especially rapidly in cosmetic surgery. About half of what our office does was introduced in *the last five years!* We have to keep learning.

An active physician who's a leader in his field attends at least six to eight professional seminars or conferences per year. A list of these conferences should be available to patients, ideally in the waiting room.

Shop Around

Cosmetic surgeons can be found in all kinds of places. Ads in your local paper or on radio are a place to start if you don't have a personal referral. However, a doctor with a national chain of clinics advertised on late night TV may be too commercial and too busy to give you the best personal care.

I suggest having consultations with at least two or three physicians, using the guidelines in this chapter to help make your decision. Although some doctors charge for these initial visits, this is less common as the field becomes more competitive.

How to React to Badmouthing and Puffery

Several of the national hair transplantation chains and at least one specialty board have taken aggressive positions about the incompetence of other physicians (badmouthing). You may also encounter individuals claiming that they are the absolute best (puffery). Unfortunately there seems to be more of this behavior in cosmetic surgery than other medical fields. It is extremely unprofessional and violates medical ethics.

Physicians are trained early in medical school to respect other doctors and not to criticize their colleagues. We are a select group who've worked very hard for our positions. Most of us understand that criticizing other doctors destroys the trust of patients for the entire medical delivery team. If you encounter badmouthing, ask yourself who it reflects on. As Shakespeare said, "The fragrance of the rose lingers on the hand that casts it." Other kinds of smells linger too.

Puffery is not as bad (we doctors are full of ourselves as you well know), but it is also unprofessional. Medical knowledge is widely spread through journals and training, and any individual or any group who claims they're the "best and only" should be tried and convicted of total egomania.

Insurance Billing for Cosmetic Procedures is Fraud

And both the doctor and the patient could go to jail! Be wary of a "deal" to do cosmetic surgery along with another medical procedure for which the insurance is billed. A few procedures, such as some breast reconstruction for overly large breasts and functional nose and eyelid work, are insurance reimbursed. Remember that you, as well as the physician, have a relationship with the insurance company, and *you* are responsible for keeping that relationship as ethical as possible.

General Anesthetics and Facility Certification

Almost all the procedures discussed in this book can be done under the new local anesthetic combinations, usually with the help of some relaxation medicines. I believe that some of these procedures, such as liposuction, *cannot* be done as accurately under general anesthesia. So ask if you will need a tube in your throat to help you breathe (and ask about the extra charges for an anesthesiologist). It may not be necessary.

Your doctor should operate in a facility that is approved by a regulatory agency. "State approved," "Medicare approved," and "AAAHC approved" are all acceptable. In some states, such as California, it is actually illegal to inject mind-altering drugs in an uncertified facility. The certificate of approval should be posted in the waiting room, so ask to see it.

Price Does Not Relate to Quality

The highest fees do not necessarily relate to the best results. When assessing fees, the factors to consider include the doctor's experience, the size of his practice, and even the location of his office. Some doctors may discount their fees for procedures in which they lack experience. They do this to attract as many new patients as possible so they can acquire the experience they need. Be sure to ask about the number of specific procedures your doctor has done (see Be Procedure Specific above).

Consider the Aesthetics of the Office

Cosmetic surgery is art, and the cosmetic surgeon's artistry is reflected in the visual qualities of his office.

If the decor is 20 years out of style, if furniture is positioned haphazardly, if things looks disorganized, if the color scheme is irritating or there's no art on the walls, then this may be an indication that the doctor doesn't have much aesthetic sense. You may not want him sculpting your hips, re-designing your eyelids or deciding where to position transplanted hair on your head.

This may also apply to the way the doctor and his staff present themselves *visually.* How do they dress? Are they well groomed? Do the staff areas and consultation rooms look organized, well-designed, and clean?

It may sound like a stretch, but it's all part of the overall feeling.

Liposuction:
The Truth about Fat

   The new liposuction dominates modern cosmetic surgery as the most commonly performed procedure, with possibly the highest satisfaction rate.

   The old surgeries for fat and skin removal are outdated and generally produce inferior results compared to skilled liposuction.

   Recovery is usually pretty easy, with most people back to work in just a few days.

   Liposuction isn't a surgical cure for overeating, but is useful in the treatment of overweight people along with exercise and diet.

   Contrary to popular belief, fat can return to the treated areas.

According to the American Academy of Cosmetic Surgery, about 300,000 people a year had liposuction in the mid 1990's. This is several times the total in 1990, and the numbers are growing faster each year. Liposuction is chosen by all ages and all types of people: men, women, models and actors, teenagers, and athletes. Some men even use it to produce "washboard abs," the sculptured abdominal muscles favored by body builders.

The liposuction procedure has changed dramatically since it was first introduced in 1979. What began as a high-risk surgery requiring routine blood transfusions and often a lengthy hospital stay has evolved into a simpler procedure performed in an outpatient surgery center. In the early days, patients were hospitalized for up to seven days. General anesthesia was used (which itself presented some risk), bleeding was often heavy, post-operative pain was excruciating, and bruising lasted for many weeks. Patients often stayed in bed for several weeks. With all that in mind, added to all of the negative media reports, popular opinion held that liposuction was a bizarre, complicated and expensive procedure.

Modern liposuction, by comparison, is completely different. It is usually virtually painless. Bleeding, infection and other complications are rare. Unfortunately, many of the old myths still live on, and realistic information is hard to come by. Let's look at the differences between today's procedures and yesterday's:

Old Style Liposuction	Modern Liposuction
Hospitalization up to seven days	A two- to five-hour procedure in an outpatient surgery center
General anesthetic	Local anesthetic
Blood transfusion often required	Little or no blood loss
Maximum of two quarts of fat removed	Sometimes 10 liters of fat or more can be removed
Incisions $1/2$ to one inch in length	Incisions as small as $1/8$ inch in length
Scarring at incision site	Little or no scarring in most cases
Excessive bruising	Mild, temporary bruising
Bed rest often needed	No bed rest generally needed
Return to normal activity in two to four weeks	Return to normal activity in two to five days
"Touch-up" procedures often needed	"Touch-up" procedures needed infrequently

Liposuction vs. "Tummy Tuck"

The "Tummy Tuck" is the old way to improve saggy "pot bellies." The surgeon would take the saggy skin of the lower abdomen and cut a big "smile" incision from hip to hip, remove the skin and fat underneath, and sew it all up. *This is major invasive surgery.* There are significant chances for infection, skin death and more serious problems. I don't want to give the impression that this sort of thing can never happen with liposuction, but it is exceedingly rare.

Tummy tuck patients generally can't walk upright without pain for three to six weeks. Additionally, most tummy tucks produce unacceptable scarring. A patient who was ashamed to show his belly before because it hung down is still ashamed of the area afterwards because of the one- or two-foot-long scar. The "belly button" often has to be repositioned, and this frequently looks strange. The contours are not always very natural. From the side, the profile shows a very flat abdomen, while from the front, the hips may be too big. And if weight gain occurs after the surgery, odd effects may result. Frequently, it is impossible to sew the skin together at the ends of the incision properly, and a "dog-ear" (this really is the medical term) occurs, where a strange little pouch of fat and skin is left on each hip.

Most "pot bellies" can be treated with liposuction alone. If properly done, the liposuction shrinks the skin and results in a reasonably good lower abdomen shape, but this requires an experienced surgeon. Sometimes the skin texture is altered, but it's generally better than taking a chance with the many problems mentioned above.

How to Prepare for Liposuction

How many times have you stood in front of the mirror wishing that you could simply remove fat from your body by some miraculous, magical process? Before the 1980s, such an idea seemed ridiculous. Now, it's not only possible, but it's usually painless, and can produce spectacular results.

But it's not magic. A physician's primary responsibility is to let patients know that liposuction is not about weight reduction. It's about reshaping and contouring the body. In cases where large quantities of fat are removed, weight reduction does occur. And although some doctors do use liposuction as an additional therapy for overweight patients, it's best not to go into it with an eye toward losing pounds. When we work with overweight patients in our office, we like to know that they have some history of attempting to control their weight with diet and exercise. The ones who get the best results are those who demonstrate a willingness to continue that commitment even after liposuction. Counseling overweight patients on diet, exercise, and a healthy lifestyle is important before making a commitment to surgery.

The Truth About Fat

One myth that keeps many people in the dark about liposuction is that fat will never return to the treated areas. Experience has shown us that the fat can indeed come back to some degree if the patient gains weight. However, most patients maintain an improved and more proportional shape, even if they do gain some weight after having liposuction.

By the time we reach physical maturity, we have a fixed number of fat cells in our bodies. When we gain weight, those cells actually grow in size. They aren't thought to multiply; it's believed that each cell actually gets "fatter." Liposuction cuts the number of fat cells in a local area of the body, but whatever cells remain can still expand if you gain weight. If, after you've had lipo, you eat improperly without exercising, the extra calories always find a home. Tightness created by the local healing process may prevent the fat from returning to the liposuctioned areas to some degree. If you really lose control of yourself and gain a lot of weight, areas that were not treated, such as face, arms, buttocks, neck or breasts, can balloon.

For those with weight problems to begin with, I cannot emphasize enough how important it is to watch the diet and stick to an exercise program after liposuction. Patients who just have small areas suctioned do not need to diet or change their exercise to look great. Liposuction is a wonderful procedure to be sure, *but it is not a surgical cure for bad eating habits or an alternative to keeping fit.*

Your Expectations

It's important to have realistic expectations about results. Outcomes are age-related, and they are also related to the shape you're in when you start out. For example, if you're a 26-year-old woman in reasonable shape, you might look like a swimsuit model after liposuction. But if you're 46 years old and 50 pounds overweight, you won't get the same result. The vast majority of liposuction patients are delighted with their results in the hands of a skilled surgeon. It's not unusual to lose one to three dress sizes (depending on the areas treated and the amount of fat that's been removed), and you may need to buy a new wardrobe. But unless you look great to start with you probably won't look like this month's centerfold after the procedure. Be realistic about where you are, and where you'd like to be.

Part of the preparation for any cosmetic procedure involves talking to your spouse, children, friends and other loved ones about your plans, and preparing them for the "new you." This sounds exciting of course, but it isn't always as easy as it seems. Some of us are in relationships in which we're expected to be depressed and lack confidence in ourselves. If we change, it can upset a balance that's been a comfortable habit for years. This may apply to professional as well as to personal relationships. If you have the courage to change, a new life is always waiting for you. For many people, cosmetic surgery can be the first step.

Most people are in good enough general health to undergo liposuction, but there are some situations in which the procedure is not recommended, specifically if a patient has an unstable medical problem such as poorly controlled diabetes or heart disease. There are no known conflicts with medication other than the use of aspirin or other blood thinners or large doses of Vitamin E, all of which can lead to bleeding and a longer recovery. If you use these products in large quantities, you will be asked to discontinue them for a week before your surgery.

How It's Done

During your initial consultation, your doctor will take a good look at your body. You'll be expected to stand there in your underwear while he studies the parts of your body that you like the least; your "saddlebags," wide hips or thighs, sagging stomach or facial "jowls." Sometimes the doctor will draw on your skin to show you which areas should be slimmed down. You'll go home with markings that look like a baby has finger-painted on you. You'll also go home excited about the prospect of transforming those areas into something that makes you feel proud.

The doctor should be able to see you in three dimensions. If he just marks a circle on your lower abdomen, he is thinking in two dimensions and you may not get the result you desire. For the "torso" cases, we generally sculpt everything from the bra-line to the lower hip all the way around the body, front and back (of course, for some young, fit people this isn't necessary). Properly done, this produces a figure that looks good from every angle.

On arrive at the surgical center the morning of your procedure, you may be given a pill such as Valium® if you're nervous. Patients may also frequently be injected with a small dose of medication like Demerol® as a pain reliever. You'll then lie on the table and have your fatty areas filled with the "tumescent solution" of sterile salt water, adrenaline and anesthetic (please refer to chapter 15 to learn more about tumescent anesthetic). Patients who need larger volumes of fat removed may be given intravenous fluids.

In about 20 minutes, when the local anesthetic has taken effect, tiny openings are made in the skin surface with a small needle (you shouldn't feel a thing). These openings are made in the areas where the fat is to be removed, most often under the buttocks, on each hip, and in the navel. A thin tube called a "cannula" (the diameter of a cocktail straw or a little bigger) is then inserted through these openings directly into the fat. The fat is then sucked out through a plastic tube into a disposable container. The whole procedure is virtually painless, and depending on the quantity of fat being removed, can take anywhere from 30 minutes to five hours. An average liposuction procedure in our office removes about two to six quarts of fat.

During the procedure, you can be awake the whole time, feeling little or no discomfort, or you may prefer to sleep. Some patients enjoy chatting casually with the doctor and his staff while they're working. In our office, you can bring in a movie to watch on the VCR or listen to your favorite music. Some patients request mild sedation and are content to lie quietly listening to music and relaxing. The experience can actually be fun, and it can give you an opportunity to bond with your doctor by telling stories and using this time to get to know each other better. One British socialite came in for liposuction carrying a cup of coffee, a Walkman with headphones and blackout eye covers. She armed herself with these things because she was nervous, but 20 minutes into the surgery she removed all the parapher-nalia and entertained us with stories for three hours.

When you're finished, you'll be "wrapped up" in a dressing that stays on for about five days. Many doctors use 6X12-inch foam pads placed directly on your skin over the treated areas (one of our patients refers to them as "giant post-it notes"). On top of that, you'll have on a girdle-like garment, which holds your skin tightly and helps keep the foam pads in place.

You'll feel fine, maybe a little tired, and many patients even feel hungry immediately after their surgery. You can go home usually an hour or so later (you will need to have someone drive you home, since there may still be some medicines in your system).

When you get home, you may be sleepy and want to relax for the remainder of the day and evening. The next day, you'll feel sore, depending on the amount of fat that was removed, and you will probably feel a bit bound-up by the foam pads and the garment, but you should feel very little discomfort. Some patients say they feel as though they'd spent the whole day doing sit-ups with an over-zealous trainer. Moving from one position to another seems to increase the discomfort. The third day is usually the worst. Then things begin to improve.

Recovery

We advise our patients to do whatever activity they can do comfortably. On the second day you can walk around the house or go out for an errand or two. By the third or the fourth day, you may return to work if you want. You should be able to resume all your normal activities, except for strenuous exercise or heavy lifting (no kick boxing for five weeks!). Some larger cases, or older patients may have some fatigue for a week or longer.

No wetting of the areas liposuctioned or bandaged with the garment for the first three days. On day 3 and 4, you may shower with the garment still on (it's just too difficult to get back on if removed). After your shower, squeeze the water out of the garment and pads with towels and then blow dry them with a hair dryer using the cool setting for about 20 minutes.

During the first one to three days you'll experience some drainage from the incision site. This is inconvenient, but perfectly normal and nothing to be alarmed about. It's the excess tumescent solution leaking out, and it can be pink to red in color because it's mixed with a tiny bit of blood (total blood loss from liposuction done with tumescent anesthesia is generally only a few tablespoons). Drainage will usually stop by the third to the seventh day, depending on how much fat was removed. The worst part is that it will stain your garment, but it can be cleaned with peroxide and/or a colorfast detergent. You may wish to purchase a second garment so you can wear one while laundering the other (a long-line girdle carried by most department stores will do fine. Sears has a good model).

On the fifth day you should remove the foam pads with some oil, and this is the first chance you'll have to get a glimpse of your new body. Patients are often overjoyed when they look into the mirror at this stage. There is a noticeable difference, but the best news is that it keeps getting better. Your body will be very swollen, and even though you can see your new shape, it will be somewhat camouflaged by puffiness. This gradually decreases over a couple of months, so your body will actually be changing and shrinking for the next 90 days (longer in some cases). You may also see bruising in some areas, but this will be gone in about two weeks. This is normal.

After you've stared at yourself in the mirror for a while, the garment must be put back on, and it should be worn for one to four weeks. Some people like wearing it a little longer, because it can sometimes be more comfortable with it on. It keeps the muscles and skin from moving around too much, kind of like a giant ace bandage, and this helps decrease the swelling and seems to relieve some soreness. When the garment is off, you may feel stiff and slightly sore. When it's on, the soreness may decrease dramatically.

By about the third week, you may start thinking about buying some new clothes. But hold out a little longer on the shopping spree, because the suctioned area should continue to shrink if you don't lose control of your eating. Also, some patients (especially the larger volume cases) have a kind of "grace period" after liposuction, during which their appetites actually decrease. There may be a period of three to six months in which you won't be as hungry as before, and this may contribute to weight loss. We wonder if this may be due to fat cell breakdown products from the liposuction somehow influencing the appetite response of the brain. At the same time, your body should be shrinking because of the healing process. For people who've been overweight most of their lives, it's the greatest feeling in the world.

Results

When you take the garment off permanently, you will more than likely love what you see in the mirror. You'll still be slightly swollen, but any bruising should be gone. You'll probably have lost a clothing size or two, and may continue to lose weight for the next several weeks. Younger people with healthy, elastic skin will find that their skin shrinks back into shape quickly. Older people, people who've had a lot of fat removed, or people who have gained and lost a lot of weight, take a bit longer. They may also notice that the skin which once covered a lot of fat may appear somewhat wrinkled. In time, it often shrinks into place on its own. The skin is a very plastic organ, especially in younger patients, and exercise always provides an enormous benefit.

You may find yourself buying more fashionable, sexier, form-revealing clothes, and wearing them proudly. You may also feel lighter, which improves your attitude and overall well-being. It's uncommon for the patients of an experienced surgeon to be disappointed with their results. Remember that results are relative to where you started, but generally they are dramatic, and the vast majority come out winners in relative terms. Since modern liposuction is done under tumescent anesthetic, complications which may result from general anesthesia are not an issue. Heart and respiratory problems are unlikely to occur. We've never heard of a case with proper tumescent anesthetic where a blood transfusion was needed, and infection occurs in less than one-half of one percent of cases. I won't claim that modern liposuction is risk-free, but it is very safe compared to most other surgeries.

The most significant complications we're aware of have to do with the results of the procedure itself. An unskilled or inexperienced surgeon may not do as good a job of "sculpting" the body, possibly leaving uneven areas or lumpiness where fat hasn't been removed properly. Some people will have some lumps and unevenness even with the best of care. Repairing a bad liposuction job rarely produces as good a result as doing it properly the first time, so choosing a surgeon who's done many, many cases is the safest bet.

If you take good care of your new body by exercising and eating right, it can be maintained for many years. If you don't stay fit and if you gain weight, you won't be happy.

---

౬ Patient Stories ౬

Barbara , age 50

No one ever knew I was a size larger on the bottom than on the top because I always wore big, loose shirts. I never took my jacket off when wearing my flight attendant uniform, except to put on my in-flight smock. I did everything I could to hide my wide hips. When I went shopping for clothes, sales people would say, "My, you're deceiving!" My thin, long neck, thin face and arms, along with long jackets gave the illusion that I was thin. I was an expert at "dressing thin."

I spoke with a few surgeons about liposuction, but never really felt safe with any of them until I met my doctor. He was able to see my flaws the same way I saw them, almost with an artist's eye. My surgery was actually fun. A couple of times during the procedure he asked me to get off the table and look at myself in the mirror so we could "fine tune" the sculpturing of my body. The experience changed my life. I now wear jeans with shirts tucked in! I never thought I'd be able to do that.

Charlene, age 43

I've always had a very healthy diet — very little meat or cheese, and almost no sweets at all. No

---

peanut butter, no junk food, and no sugary drinks. I also exercised on my Nordic Track three times a week. But for some reason, I couldn't change my large, flabby thighs, sagging tummy, and wide hips. It's genetic I guess, but nothing could fix it.

The doctor I decided to work with was very encouraging, and when I had the surgery, it was in many ways the happiest day of my life. I couldn't believe the difference in my shape. I went from size 12 to a size 8. It's been two years, and I've gained some weight back because I haven't been exercising. But I still look better than I could have ever hoped to look.

Cynthia, age 36

After I had a baby, I really needed a boost of self esteem because I was so unhappy with the way my body looked. A friend referred me to her doctor after she'd had liposuction. And she really looked good.

During my initial consult, I felt very relaxed with the office staff and the atmosphere of the place. I had the lipo, and it's the best thing that's happened to me in a long time. I'd recommend it to anyone. It's been seven months, and I get inspired every time I look at my new, flat stomach, so I do sit ups religiously.

Janice, age 45

I've been dieting my whole life. I was a chunky kid, and I've always been big, but even though I'm shapely and evenly distributed, my stomach and mid-section have always been out of control.

I started out having lipo on my thighs only, because I was quite large and didn't want to do too much at once. I had 6.5 liters of fat removed just from my thighs. I was only out of work for four days. I did it on a Thursday and was back to work on Monday.

I'm very pleased with the results. In fact, I think the whole thing's been amazing. So far, the fat has not come back, and although I'm on the road a lot and it's hard to exercise, I'm still in the lower sizes after nine months.

When I first took the foam pads off and looked in the mirror, I saw a body that I'd never seen before. I had a waist! To me, I looked like Barbie.

Kate, age 49

My 18-year-old daughter had very rounded hips which protruded a lot. It was genetic, and although she exercised and ate right, she couldn't get rid of the fat. I'd been looking around for a liposuction doctor, and after interviewing a few, we made our choice.

My daughter's results were just fabulous. I'm so happy to see her wearing clothes that she loves, and it really helped her self-esteem. I liked her results so much that I decided to do it myself, to have liposuction on my stomach. I'd had a Cesarean, and I had that scar with the sagging on both sides. The doctor just evened the whole thing out. And now I have a flat stomach *and* a waistline. *During her liposuction, Kate also had fat transplanted into her face and buttocks. Please see chapter 9 for details about this procedure.*

Dr. Yoho's Philosophy of Facial Rejuvenation

෨ *The best results are obtained by doing several procedures at once, as opposed to concentrating on just one isolated flaw.*

෨ *A face lift isn't the only solution for most facial problems. Other techniques are often more appropriate, and therapy should be individualized.*

My patients often point to one little facial problem and say, "Doctor, if you could just get rid of these little wrinkles (or little saggy area, or acne scar), I'll be very happy with myself and feel better." I've got to tell you, it just ain't so.

I *can* work on just one little facial problem, and I do sometimes. But the patient may not be terribly impressed with the result. The real drama of the cosmetic surgeon's art is most evident when working on *many little defects* to produce the ultimately improved *whole*. Details as small as the removal of a mole can have a much more powerful effect when it's done in combination with other procedures.

Also, when a patient looks in the mirror and is unhappy with the way he or she looks, the first thing that traditionally comes to mind is, "I need a face lift." Most patients aren't sophisticated enough to understand that this isn't the answer to every problem. A face lift may improve deep wrinkles and sagginess, but will do almost nothing for texture and pigment problems, which are often more prominent. These can be more effectively treated with a laser peel or creams. Color changes, enlarged pores due to aging, and sun-damaged skin can be improved with relatively inexpensive therapies that patients can apply themselves. But most importantly, with age, the skin loses the fat "foundation" of the face. The best way to address this is often to replace the lost fat. I'll describe this in chapter 9, which describes fat transplantation.

I believe that a proper laser peel which evenly "shrinks the skin to fit," combined with proper fat replacement to build out the underlying structures, makes the "cut and sew" face lift obsolete in many cases. The results are just so much more dramatic and natural when the key cosmetic elements of fat loss and texture are properly addressed, as opposed to stretching and cutting. Face lifts can be great, but we think they are often best for the over 65-year-old age group. And even then we'd like you to consider the newer techniques, because they often work better.

We want to emphasize that everyone has his or her own individual facial rejuvenation problem, depending on age, sex, ethnic origin, previous sun exposure, skin pigment and other factors. A "one size fits all" approach guarantees mediocre results. Ultimately, you'll be happier with a combination of procedures that fits you. Depending on your face, fat transplantation, laser peeling, cream treatments, selective liposuction, face-lifting, and/or an "eyelid lift" can be used in some combination to make you look your best.

Facial Laser Peel

🐪 *Carbon dioxide (CO_2) and Erbium laser peels have replaced acid (chemical) peeling and dermabrasion as the safest, most effective facial resurfacing procedures today.*

🐪 *Light TCA peels are safe and good for minor pigment color improvement and a freshening effect.*

🐪 *Wrinkles respond better than scars.*

🐪 *The skin of the treated area shrinks to some degree.*

🐪 *The procedure can be done by skilled practitioners under local anesthetic.*

🐪 *Recovery is irritating but not generally painful, with a relatively low chance of complications.*

The American Academy of Cosmetic Surgeons reports that 72 percent of people who consult cosmetic surgeons do so because they're interested in facial work. The reason is simple — the face is the most visible part of the body. Whether we like it or not, we're judged by first impressions, and our faces tell the stories of our lives. In 1996, over half a million individuals had some kind of facial cosmetic surgery, some involving a hospital stay and many using general anesthesia.

Facial laser peeling, by contrast, can be done in one afternoon in a doctor's office. Local anesthesia can be used if the doctor is an expert in the use of tumescent anesthesia (see chapter 15 for more information on tumescent anesthesia). The results are generally excellent, and the recovery is quite manageable.

Patients desire facial laser peels for a variety of reasons: most often for wrinkles, acne scarring, discoloration, and other skin imperfections. Most of our patients choose to treat the entire face, but some have work done only around the eyes or the mouth. Either way, if done skillfully, laser peeling can produce remarkable improvements.

In the "old days" before laser peels came into common use, two techniques were used instead; "dermabrasion" and "chemical" or "acid" peeling. Although these procedures are still used today, they produce more frequent complications, including scarring and/or permanent changes in skin color. These things can happen with a laser peel, but it's rare.

Dermabrasion involves using a tiny electric sander which revolves at a very high speed, and literally "sands" the surface of the skin. A good surgeon can "rub out" wrinkles or acne scars to an even plane, but it requires a lot more skill than the laser, and scarring or uneven results are more common. Dermabrasion also produces a lot of bleeding. It's been said in some medical texts that 50 percent of dermabrasion patients wish they'd never had the procedure.

Acid peeling is the chemical version of the same idea. Rather than sanding the skin surface, one of two acids — phenol or trichloracetic (TCA) — is applied to produce a deep, hopefully even, injury to the old skin. Phenol produces a lot of wrinkle shrinkage, but also produces permanent color loss *in virtually every case*. Patients often end up with a white cast to their faces, which will need to be covered up with make-up. Generally this is acceptable only in elderly patients.

When enough TCA (40 to 50 percent strength) is applied to produce significant wrinkle shrinkage and deep penetration, there is at least a three to five percent chance of scarring. When it penetrates too deep, scarring occurs. No one can accurately predict how this more powerful TCA will penetrate the skin. In my opinion, this makes deep TCA peeling unacceptable.

Superficial TCA peeling, however, is an excellent technique. Low concentrations of TCA are placed on the face, producing skin changes that are obvious during the application process but are different from the deep TCA peel. This is also good for texture improvement. Recovery time for this lighter peel may only be four to five days, but deep wrinkles are not affected. Fruit acid, such as 40 to 70 percent Glycolic acid, is also being used in a similar fashion as the light (20 to 25 percent) TCA peeling.

By 1994, laser technology had entered the mainstream as a treatment to replace dermabrasion and chemical peels. Not every doctor has adopted the new technology. Laser equipment is very expensive — more than $100,000 for a state-of-the-art setup — and special training is required. But the medical community's feeling overall is that laser peeling is more predictable and complication-free than the other techniques.

How to Prepare for Facial Laser Surgery

Prior to facial laser surgery, some patients are asked to treat their faces with Retin A® and/or skin bleaches or creams for two to four weeks. Because dark skinned people can sometimes darken further after the procedure, they are frequently advised to treat their skin before surgery to prevent this. We also require our patients to take an anti-viral medication such as

Valtrex® or Acyclovir® to prevent cold sores, which can be stimulated by the treatment. Cold sores can spread all over the face and cause scarring if they occur after treatment when the skin is raw. You also don't want to undergo a surgical procedure if you are ill or if you have unstable medical problems. Your doctor will counsel you about any limitations.

I believe that preparing for your recovery is the most important element to consider when it comes to facial laser peeling. Patients should be given an accurate picture of what to expect during this period, because frankly, a newly peeled face is not a pretty sight. Most patients choose to stay in the house for a week or two after the procedure, as their faces are either bandaged, or if exposed, raw and swollen. So plan to take adequate time off from work, and don't book any important social engagements until at least two weeks after your laser peel. Let your family and friends know what to expect.

How It's Done

When you arrive at your doctor's office, you'll get your picture taken (before and after photos are *very* important). Then you'll be given a sedative, and while you're relaxing, the doctor may draw on your face to mark the areas to be treated. Your face will then be washed with an antiseptic solution and the tumescent solution will be injected with a tiny needle to numb the face. If the doctor is *not* using tumescent, he may alternatively have an anesthesiologist put you to sleep.

By the time the doctor begins working with the laser tool, you shouldn't feel anything at all. The laser "zaps" small areas on the face as the doctor moves carefully from one area to the next, treating each in turn, making sure to blend everything evenly. In the past, lasers could only work on very small spots, about an eighth of an inch at a time. But now, the technology has improved to the point where we can "laser" spots about 1.5 centimeters (about two-thirds of an inch) in diameter, using a laser pattern generator. This is an important advance, because working with larger spots produces a much more even effect.

The laser doesn't actually burn the skin, because there's very little heat transfer involved. Instead, it *vaporizes* the skin surface by making the water boil inside the skin. During the process, the treated skin changes in a way that allows the doctor to wipe off the top layers with a wet gauze pad. With each zap of the laser, the doctor can see new, fresh skin appear. Almost no bleeding occurs. Each laser zap lasts a fraction of a second, and if you're awake (but sleepy) during the procedure, you'll hear it working — zip, zip, zip — and you may hear the doctor and staff talking and working around you. The whole process lasts about an hour when the pattern generator lasers are used.

Recovery

When the procedure is finished, you may be feeling drugged, and you'll need someone to drive you home. When you get there, you may want to sleep for a few hours until the drugs work their way out of your system. The next morning you'll generally feel normal.

You'll often leave the doctor's office with a dressing on your face or sometimes a layer of Vaseline® on your skin. There are many different schools of thought about dressings, and doctors are continually learning more about which are most effective. I believe that dressings are important for recovery from a peel deep enough to remove wrinkles effectively. The depth of the treatment is proportional to the risk, the recovery and the results. For very deep peels, it's helpful to leave dressings in place for about five days (some doctors do deep peels without dressings, but I don't feel this is as safe). A clear benefit is that patients have virtually no pain when modern full-face dressings are used for a full five days. They describe their dressings as annoying but not painful. For lighter peels used to treat more minor facial problems, a dressing may be removed sooner or may not be needed at all.

Our deep-peel patients leave the office with their faces wrapped like a mummy or "the invisible man." The eyes and lips are exposed, and may swell, and they look very strange at first. One patient's four-year-old son became very frightened when his mom returned home with her face bandaged. He wouldn't let her near him until her face normalized. He even had nightmares. Depending on the depth of your laser peel, you might want to make arrangements to have very young children stay at Grandma's for a few days, or prepare them well for the event.

Pain just isn't a big issue with most laser peel recoveries when the full face dressing is used. Some people have a slight burning sensation (if you are having much pain, get in to see the doctor right away — you may be having a cold sore outbreak which can cause scarring). Others have itching, and special creams may be used to relieve this. The most irritating thing is the night-and-day facial wrap and the strange feeling of your swollen face. For the first day or two, it will help to ice your face several times a day for ten to twenty minutes with a damp washcloth (or the dressing) between the skin and the ice.

You may also find that the swelling (and sometimes the dressing) makes it difficult to move your mouth comfortably for the first couple of days. Some people lose a little weight because they don't eat much. When the dressing is removed, your face will be red and still swollen. Your skin will feel dry and tight, and you should keep it lubricated with whatever cream your doctor recommends.

The best path to a speedy recovery is by way of the hyperbaric chamber (see chapter 17 for a complete explanation of how the hyperbaric chamber works). It's an expensive and high-tech piece of equipment sometimes found in hospitals for use with seriously ill patients, such as burn victims. Today, there are only a few places in the United States where facilities other than hospitals have hyperbaric chambers, but this will likely change soon. The chamber may have the potential to cut healing time almost in half, and is remarkably effective on laser peels.

Depending on the depth of your laser peel, you can expect to look presentable with makeup in one to two weeks. During the second and third weeks, the swelling decreases, but redness remains. Don't expect to lose all the redness for several months. You may also experience some temporary darkening, which can be treated with bleaching creams and should disappear in time.

Results

Just as in your recovery, your results are related to the depth of the peel. It's not recommended for a doctor to go too deep in one session, so for some very wrinkled faces or deep acne scars, patients may require a second procedure to get the best results. People who smoke tend to have deeper lines around their lips and may require a deeper laser peel. Sometimes there are fine details which aren't noticeable until after healing is complete, and these patients may return for an additional laser treatment. It's simple to "touch up" a small area. The vast majority of the patients in our office are delighted with their results.

Your skin should look softer, younger and smoother. Wrinkle removal can be very dramatic. With deeper peels, the new skin will "shrink to fit" your face. Healing of human injuries is accomplished by shrinkage of the tissue, and what the laser does is provide a careful "injury" to the skin. Brown spots generally disappear. Patients are usually asked to use light moisturizers for at least a month. Occasionally, acne breakouts can occur as a result of this at one to three months, but it can be treated by decreasing the lubricants and possibly prescribing antibiotics.

๛ Patient Stories ๕

Chanelle, age 45 — Full face laser

I'm one of those women who spent my entire youth frying my skin in the sun. In my 20s, I'd spend five or six hours a day at the beach several times a week, lying on the sand with my face to the sun, working on that perfect tan. As I got older and heard about the damage this could do, I simply ignored all that and went on with my life as a sun worshipper. But when I turned 40, the damage was too obvious to ignore.

I had a facial laser peel and couldn't believe the difference in my skin. The little wrinkles pretty much disappeared, especially around my eyes, and my whole face looked smoother, like brand-new skin had grown there.

Sarah, age 71 — Full face laser

I haven't been happy with the look of my skin for many years. I had liver spots, wrinkles, and everything else that comes with age. Two years ago I lost a son, and all that pain and sorrow did something to my face. I didn't want to look sad anymore. I decided after research that the laser peel was my best option. I had my procedure five weeks ago. Today, as I'm healing, my face looks like it has a bad sunburn, but I can really see a difference. It really didn't change my face. It just made me look calmer. Softer. It's very subtle.

Angela, age 74 — Full face laser

My daughter had it done last year. She was 47. When my husband saw her results, it gave him the courage to tell me how much the bags under my eyes had been bothering him all these years. So about six months ago, I had a laser peel done. Even though I did it to please him, I'm so happy that I did it, because I love the way I look. My husband raves about it to anyone who'll listen. When I was young, people didn't talk about these things. Nowadays, we admire people for doing something like this.

Eyelid Reconstruction

🗷 *Baggy eyelids can now be improved with the laser instead of a scalpel, with a shorter recovery. The two to three weeks of bruising that was common after an eyelid surgery using a scalpel is rare when laser is used.*

🗷 *Lower eyelids are now treated with a laser incision **inside** the lower eyelid, so healing is easier and there is no visible scar.*

🗷 *The laser is also used to shrink the skin on the outside of the eyelids to produce smooth skin in the manner of a laser peel.*

Eyelid surgery — or "blepharoplasty" — is a relatively simple surgery with a very high satisfaction rate. Older people tend to seek help more often than younger people, as the fat and skin around their eyes begins to sag. But if droopy eyelids are characteristic in your family, blepharoplasty may be helpful regardless of your age. Patients as young as 30 have told me that they were prompted to seek surgery after years of hearing friends say, "You look so tired. Are you OK?"

Blepharoplasty is popular with men as well as women, particularly male executives who have to compete in a job market constantly being infiltrated by younger men. They want to erase the signs of stress that have accumulated on their faces over the years by softening the look of their skin, erasing some of their wrinkles, and eliminating a good portion of the "bags" of fat that have accumulated under the eyes. The goal is a younger overall look, and patients are usually exceedingly satisfied.

Although blepharoplasty has traditionally been performed with a knife, scalpel incisions more frequently cause bleeding, often leaving patients with black and blue eyes for weeks. When laser technology became popular in the mid 1990s, the procedure became easier and safer. Because the laser seals off blood vessels, there is usually no bruising, since bruising is a result of bleeding. The laser is also used to resurface the skin of the eyelids and "crow's feet," removing wrinkles and improving texture.

How It's Done

When you arrive in the doctor's office, you'll be given a mild sedative to help you relax, plus some intravenous sedation (sometimes general anesthetic is used, but this is not necessary). You'll also be given some special eye drops to numb the eyelids, and this usually prevents you from feeling the local anesthetic which is injected next. These injections are given with a tiny needle and numb the area around the eyes. During the procedure, you may be awake enough to hear the doctor's voice, but you shouldn't feel any pain or discomfort. If a laser is being used, steel eye covers are placed over the eyes to protect them. These are quite comfortable.

Blepharoplasty can be done on the upper or the lower eyelids. Let's begin by addressing the lower lid first.

Under the Eye

An incision is made into the "conjunctiva" or the inside part of the lower eyelid. In the past, blepharoplasty was done by making a small smile-like incision beneath the eyelash on the lower lid. However, an external incision like this has frequently led to complications, including bleeding, excessive bruising and something called "scleral show." This means that the lower eyelid is pulled down so far that too much sclera (the white part of the eye) shows. The external incision, whether done with a scalpel or a laser, is only done these days when there is a lot of extra skin to remove. Many doctors, particularly ophthalmologists, think that this is a risky, outdated technique, and that it should virtually never be used.

Once the incision is made, fat deposits which have built up inside the lid are simply removed with the laser. Whether the procedure is done with a laser or a scalpel, stitches inside the eyelid are not necessary, and healing is perfect in the vast majority of cases.

Upper Eyelids

Many people with upper eyelid problems not only have cosmetic concerns, but may have so much excess fat and skin that the eyelid can actually drop low enough to block vision and cause fatigued eyes. The treatment for this is to remove a crescent of skin on the eyelid, along with a small amount of eyelid muscle and fat. The incision is closed with stitches.

This procedure can be done with a scalpel, as with the lower lids, but laser technology has improved the whole process tremendously for the reasons I outlined earlier. As with the lower lids, the results may be improved if a laser peel is also done on the outside of the upper lids to improve the texture.

Standards of beauty are different in different cultures, and there have been stories about Asian people having eyelid reconstruction in an attempt to "Caucasianize" their looks. While this may be true for a handful of individuals, most patients want their natural looks enhanced rather than changed. Asians generally like a low natural crease in their eyelids. About 40 percent have never had the kind of crease they desire, and we can create it for them. Also, when Asian people age, that crease can sometimes drop down so far that it actually sits right on top of the eyelash line. We don't want to make high creases like a Caucasian or a shape reminiscent of a Disney character, which is totally unnatural for Asians. We just raise slightly and sharpen the natural crease, and form a taper down toward the nose area.

Recovery

When the procedure is finished, you may feel sleepy due to the medications, and the usual office policy requires that you have someone drive you home. You'll possibly feel drowsy for the rest of the day and evening depending on how much medication you were given.

Because we often do a laser peel on the lower eyelids of our blepharoplasty patients, this recovery is similar to the facial laser peel recovery, but limited to the area around the eyes (please see chapter 5 for information on facial laser peeling). Usually the lower lids just get ointment and no dressing.

You may feel a slight burning sensation around the peeled areas, but this can be relieved by applying ice with a wet washcloth between the ice and the skin. Discomfort only lasts a day or two. If your upper eyelids were treated, you'll have seven to 15 tiny stitches in the eyelid crease. On the lower lids, there are generally no stitches if the incision was made inside.

There is virtually no pain during the recovery period, but because your eyelids are swollen and the skin has been stretched, you may experience some difficulty closing your eyes properly for several days or, in some instances, several weeks. In rare cases, patients have trouble sleeping in the beginning because their eyes don't close correctly. This should pass in time and can be relieved by using lubricating eye drops and/or sleeping with an eye shade. Occasionally the doctor may prescribe stretching exercises for your eyelid skin.

Since your eyes will be swollen from the surgery, and your skin will look red and raw from the laser peel, you might not want to go anywhere for the first few days. Some people are able to return to work in one to two days, and others opt to stay out longer. The redness from the laser peel will usually last from one to two months, and it will look like a sunburn, but it will gradually fade away. During the first few weeks you may want to wear sunglasses. After new skin has grown back in one to two weeks, any remaining redness or temporary discoloration can be covered with makeup. In some cases color changes need to be treated with bleaching creams.

Results

The upper eyelid stitches will be removed anywhere from three to ten days after surgery. If the incision was made with a scalpel, less healing time is needed. The incision line is generally formed in the crease of the lid, so when your eyes are open, it is usually invisible. On the lower lids, if the incisions were made inside the lid, there should be no visible trace at all.

Complications are very rare. Blindness occurs in one of about 40,000 cases when a scalpel is used, and this happens because of bleeding behind the eye, but it is exceedingly unlikely with the laser. The laser simply creates less bleeding. Of course, because steel eye shields are used, there is virtually no chance of the laser hitting the eye itself and causing problems. Other possible complications include eyelid asymmetry, small cysts occurring along the top eyelid suture line, dry eyes, and uneven patches of fat remaining in the treated areas. But all of these complications are quite rare, and when they do occur, they are often corrected with minor surgery that in most instances doesn't require sedation or relaxation medicines. Overall, the satisfaction rate is very high with blepharoplasty.

Patients usually feel and look healthier and younger. Often, after excess fat has been removed, they can actually open their eyes more comfortably than before (this is especially true for older patients). Blepharoplasty also seems to reduce eye fatigue for people who find it difficult to keep their eyes open at night when they're tired. It also allows women to use makeup more efficiently, because the upper eyelid becomes a better platform for it. The overall effect is generally quite impressive, creating a more youthful, relaxed look.

ཞ Patient Stories ℘

Judy, age 45

I had my eyelids "done" when I had my facial laser peel. The doctor had explained to me about how it would remove the little pockets of fat on my upper eyelids, and for days before the surgery, I'd look in the mirror, pulling my eyelids up and trying imagine what it would look like. The real thing was much better than I'd imagined. My eyes look more open. More aware. Overall, I look less tired. I've always liked my eyes, but now, I think they're just incredible.

Jim, age 48

Everyone in my family has droopy looking eyes. You can tell we're from the same family because our eyes are so similar. When I was in my 20s, people commented about how tired or how sad I looked. I wasn't tired or sad. I just had these droopy eyes.

I finally did something about it five years ago, and it was the best money I ever spent. It lifted my eyes up and made me look more awake. Nobody since then has said anything about how tired I look. When I look at my mother and my brother now, I can see my former eyes on their faces. I wish they would consider having their eyelids improved too.

Face Lifts

7

The information here was contributed by my colleague, Dr. Mani Nambiar.

ƥ Face lifting works best for elderly people with very loose baggy skin on their faces. I don't think it is the best technique for younger people. It certainly isn't a cure-all for every facial problem.

ƥ *A long incision around the whole face is necessary, and the skin around the entire face is pulled back and sewn into place at the edge.*

Although facial liposuction, laser peeling and fat transplantation are the most contemporary methods for treating aging facial skin, there are always cases in which a traditional surgical face lift can provide added benefits. While facial liposuction and laser peeling can tighten the face, these procedures can be less effective than a face lift if there is a very large amount of excess skin. In some cases, a face lift has the potential to create a longer-lasting effect than a laser peel or fat transplant.

How to Prepare

Once you've decided to have surgery, preoperative pictures will be taken. Aspirin and vitamin E must be discontinued a week or so prior to the procedure, because they may contribute to bleeding. If you smoke, be warned. Many doctors will not do face lifts on smokers, and all encourage quitting before this surgery.

After a history, physical exam, and blood tests are taken, patients are instructed to clean the face and hair with an antibacterial soap and shampoo before surgery. Antibiotics are usually taken the day before the procedure.

Proper selection of the right patient is very important for face lifts, and patients with prominent facial bones are ideal candidates. A combination of several surgical procedures may be most beneficial, and these may include liposuction, fat transfer, laser, or chin and cheek implants, depending the patient's needs. Some doctors do face lifts for younger patients these days because they believe the results last longer when the skin is more elastic.

Unlike many of the other procedures we've discussed, a face lift is more serious surgery because it involves a long cut into the skin. A line is cut from in front of one ear, ending behind the other ear (honest — the incision is over a foot long). The skin is then loosened, pulled upwards toward the scalp line, and stitched into place. Because so much cutting is involved, the recovery is different than it is for other facial procedures. There is a higher risk of bleeding and infection with face lifts, and the results are more variable, depending on the elasticity of the skin and the skill of the surgeon. Be sure your doctor thoroughly explains the procedure, the recovery, and the risks, and be sure you become familiar with alternatives such as laser peeling or fat implantation.

As is the case with all facial surgery, you're going to look bruised and swollen for several weeks. There will be a long, running stitch or staples from in front of your ear all the way to the back and into the hair line, so be prepared to look a little strange for a while.

Many patients stay at home for a week or two, until their faces begin to look normal again, while others choose to wear sunglasses and maybe a scarf over their faces to go about their daily lives. It depends on your comfort level.

Finally, arrange for someone to accompany you to the doctor's office, because you'll need someone to drive you home while the medications are still in your system.

How It's Done

When you arrive at the doctor's office, you'll be given a sedative to relax you, and then you will be injected with tumescent anesthesia if this is used (please see chapter 15 for a description of tumescent anesthesia). Most face lifts are done under general anesthesia, but we prefer tumescent because there's less bleeding during the procedure, less bruising, and a shorter recovery later on. By the time surgery begins, you shouldn't be feeling any discomfort at all. You may be asleep or just slightly awake in a "Twilight Sleep."

Today, careful liposuction is often performed on fatty areas of the face and neck before the rest of the procedure starts. Then, the long incision is made around the ears and into the scalp. Sometimes only the part around the ear is treated, depending on the looseness of the skin. But if the whole operation is done, the skin of nearly the entire face and neck is lifted up from its attachments with instruments or the surgeon's fingers. The excess skin all around the sides of the face is then cut off. Stitches or staples are next placed all around the edges of the face. In some cases, a deeper layer of tissue located underneath the surface layer may also be tightened with permanent sutures. A foam dressing is applied. This is the traditional face lift.

A newer technique — called a "deep plane" face lift — has recently been introduced. This involves going deeper into the face, underneath the muscle, and pulling the muscle up along with the skin to make the lift last longer. This may help the face to hold up better, and may produce a longer lasting effect. The risks for this procedure are higher than they are for a classic face lift.

Some doctors choose to laser peel the surface of the face on the day the face lift is performed, to improve the skin's overall texture.

Recovery

When you leave the doctor's office, your face will be completely bandaged. You'll feel groggy, but there is surprisingly little pain. The bandage needs to remain on until you return to the doctor's office, usually in one to three days. At this point, the doctor will be checking to see if there has been any bleeding under the skin, clotting or excessive swelling (if you've also had a laser peel, see chapter 5 for information on laser peel recovery). Postoperative pain isn't usually a big issue with traditional face lifts, but the doctor should supply appropriate medication. If the deeper face lift was performed, there may be more pain.

It might be difficult to move your eyes and mouth due to the tightness of the skin and the swelling, so don't plan on eating or talking too much for the first five to seven days. The skin will loosen up a bit as it heals, and the swelling will decrease day by day. You'll begin to see your new face almost immediately.

The stitches can be removed in about 10 days. The incision line really isn't very visible on most people because their hair covers it. You may experience bruising around the incision area, and possibly around the eyes and chin. This occurs because the skin has been aggressively manipulated, and bruising is normal. It rarely lasts more than three weeks (occasionally bleeding under the skin occurs, and may delay recovery). Most of the swelling should be gone at the end of the first month.

Results

When done properly, the results of a face lift can be very impressive. By contrast, in the hands of a surgeon who may be inexperienced or unskilled, results can be problematic. Many of us have seen celebrities and others who've had "bad" face lifts. They look like their faces have been stretched too far, as if they are startled, or a strong wind is blowing their skin back. This is a moderately common complication.

Loss of hair at the incision site is another problem that can occur. Some patients have hair transplants to lower their hairlines enough to cover the incision, and many have to alter their hair styles permanently to conceal the thinning look or the scarring. There is usually some sort of incision mark left in front of the ears, and sometimes the scalp line incision is visible. There are scars behind the ears which usually aren't very visible, and these can possibly prohibit wearing ponytails or swept-up hair-dos. It is also possible that in time, the lifted skin will loosen up again, simply because it's going against gravity. Lifting the muscle along with the skin can address this problem, but it's not a guarantee against sagging. Younger people tend to get better results because their skin is more elastic and can hold itself up better. The doctor needs to know and understand how to delicately balance the amount of skin tension in order to get the best possible result.

ଛ Patient Stories ଷ

Anna, age 61

I'd heard that going through a face lift was a traumatic experience, and I guess in some ways it was. The scar and the bruising was pretty bad at first, and I was afraid I'd never look normal again. But it got better each day, and after a few weeks, I was completely amazed at the improvement. The scar isn't really visible, and I'm very happy with the results.

Betty, age 59

I had a face lift about five years ago because I was so unhappy with my sagging skin and facial jowls. After all this time, it still looks good. I was lucky that had a very good doctor, because I'd heard horror stories about all the things that could go wrong. The recovery was uncomfortable and difficult, but it was worth it.

Nose Reconstruction and Chin Improvement

This chapter was contributed by my colleague, Dr. Mani Nambiar.

Ȣ *When skillfully performed, "nose jobs" can enhance both breathing and appearance.*

Ȣ *The major part of the recovery takes usually less than a week.*

Ȣ *Chin implants or chin reductions are sometimes needed to create the best look.*

Reconstruction of the nose, or a "nose job," is one of the most familiar cosmetic surgeries. It was, at one time, the third most popular cosmetic surgery after liposuction and breast enhancement. However, although technology has advanced and the procedure is safer and more reliable than ever, the popularity of nose reconstruction has actually decreased in recent years. One reason is that more and more people are choosing to retain their ethnic individuality, which is often expressed predominantly in the shape of the nose.

Patients seek nose work for both cosmetic and medical reasons. "Rhinoplasty" is done to improve the patient's looks, and "septoplasty" and "turbinectomy" are commonly performed to improve breathing. All of these procedures can be done in an outpatient surgical center under local anesthetic.

Chin augmentation ("mentoplasty") or reduction ("genioplasty") is sometimes also recommended. Mentoplasty can help when a retruded or small chin tends to make a large nose appear larger on a person's face, and genioplasty can correct a larger or protrusive chin which makes a nose appear smaller. Sometimes one or the other procedure is recommended in addition to rhinoplasty, since a good nose reconstruction can appear only fair if a person's face now has a disproportionate balance to the nose, especially when viewed in profile.

How It's Done

Rhinoplasty

Two types of problems usually inspire people to call the nose doctor — a large bone or "hump" on the bridge of the nose, or an oversized, bulbous area at the tip. Most patients have concerns about their appearance for many years by the time they decide to have surgery, and usually they'll come in with a magazine picture or a photo showing the nose they'd like to have. Although we can't guarantee an exact match, we do our best, while making sure that the new nose is still appropriately related to the face.

When you arrive at the doctor's office, you'll be given a mild sedative such as Valium®, and possibly a stronger medicine like Demerol® to relax. We then inject the nose with a numbing medicine such as Xylocaine®. For nose work, we don't use tumescent anesthetic, because the fluid fills up the area so much that we can't get an accurate visual sense of what we're working on. The swelling camouflages the true picture.

There are two ways in which rhinoplasty can be done. Traditionally, incisions are made inside the nostrils which are not visible from the outside. This is called a "closed" or "endonasal" rhinoplasty. Very simple instruments, similar to a file and a chisel, are inserted through the incision all the way to the bone and cartilage, which is then reshaped. You've probably heard that nose jobs require that the bones be intentionally broken. What really happens is that when the nose bones are too wide apart, in order to narrow them, they must be fractured to produce the new shape. Within five or six days, the bones will have melded together by the healing process.

To improve the shape of the nose tip, the doctor uses tiny scissors to cut away the soft tissue that forms the enlarged section. Often, the tip will need to be better defined after the soft tissue is removed, and we do this by adding extra cartilage — usually taken from the inside of the central nose (septum). This cartilage is stitched into place. This is referred to as a grafting procedure.

There's a new method practiced more and more these days in which a horizontal incision is made on the outside, on the "columella" (central part between the nostrils). This is called "open rhinoplasty." This type of incision gives the doctor an excellent view of and access to the structures of the nose, which can make for a more accurate reconstruction, but may produce more scarring. In most cases, the choice is the patient's. Be sure to discuss both options with your doctor.

Turbinectomy and Septoplasty

The medical reason for a nose job is simple — to breathe better. This can be done in several different ways. Sometimes nose repair is done to improve a crooked septum (the interior "wall" between the two nostrils). Everybody has some irregularity in the septum, because nothing in the body is perfectly straight or perfectly symmetrical. But if this deflection is extreme, it can obstruct air flow. This corrective procedure, called septoplasty, is done with the same incision and the same instruments as rhinoplasty.

Another medical reason for nose reconstruction is to help counter the long-term effects of certain allergies. Inside the nose there are small round balls of bone and soft tissue called "turbinates." People who are allergic to dust, pollen or other irritants may find that over the years, the turbinates have swollen and grown larger in response to the allergens. If the allergies are diagnosed and managed properly, the turbinates will shrink. But in cases where the allergies haven't been treated, these structures may have to be reduced surgically to increase the air passage size. This is a purely medical procedure, but often the surgeon can do a little redesigning of the nose while doing the turbinectomy.

Mentoplasty

If the chin is the only area to be treated, then the mentoplasty can usually be done under local anesthetic or with a light sedative.

Augmentation of the chin can be done in two ways. The first and notably most frequently performed way is to place contoured synthetic material made of silicone, polyethylene, or acrylic over the bone of the chin. These are called "alloplastic" materials. There are many different shapes and sizes of chin implants. The patient's cosmetic goals combined with the cosmetic surgeon's aesthetic and surgical knowledge play a part in deciding which implants to use.

The incision used to place the implant can be placed inside the mouth (intra-orally) or through the skin in areas under the chin, either way making it invisible to the casual observer. There tends to be a slightly larger incidence of infection, though, with the intra-oral route. Instruments are used to create a pocket either over or under the thick covering of the bone, or "periosteum." Under the periosteum tends to give a tighter jaw-lift with less post-operative movement of the implant. The implant is placed into the pocket and is sutured or sometimes held with micro-screws placed into the bone through the implant. A chin dressing or strap is placed and will usually remain on for a minimum of five to seven days, to help mold the chin implant in position and minimize post-operative swelling.

The second way to add to a chin is to use the patient's own bone by making a cut, sliding the chin bone forward, and securing it in position with screws and wires. This is a good method if the chin needs to be lengthened vertically as well as advanced forward. This procedure seems to be more invasive and requires more anesthetic, time, and surgical equipment. The incision is most often done intra-orally inside the lower lip to expose the bony chin. A surgical saw is then used to horizontally cut through the chin below the roots of the teeth and the nerves that come out of the jaw bone on either side that supply sensation to the skin tissue of the lower lip and chin area. The bony chin is then advanced forward and, if necessary, lengthened vertically with bone graft material, then secured into position as mentioned above. As this is a larger surgical procedure, there is some risk for injury to the nerves that supply the lip and chin, and more bleeding and post-operative swelling.

Genioplasty

Chin reduction is done by either removing bone or by performing a bone cut as described above and sliding the chin backwards.

Recovery

Nose Reconstructions

The recovery is about the same for both functional and cosmetic nose jobs. If a facial laser peel is done at the same time to even out the skin surface, the patient will have to undergo laser recovery as well (please see chapter 5 on facial laser peeling).

After your procedure, you'll leave the office wearing a splint, which must stay in place for five days. Occasionally there will be a gauze or cotton packing placed inside the nose to inhibit bleeding, and this usually remains in place for two to five days. But on day five, everything comes off, and you will actually be able to clearly see the new shape of your nose. There will be swelling, but by the third week, 70 percent of it is generally gone. In some cases there will be bruising under the eyes. This is usually minimal and temporary.

There is little or no pain during the recovery period, and most patients do not need prescription pain killers, although these are given just in case. The cotton packing is usually the most uncomfortable aspect of recovery. Some doctors have even found the packing unnecessary, because there is seldom any bleeding.

In a very few cases complications can occur, such as immediate post-operative bleeding (less than two percent), or irregularities in the shape of the nose. "Touch-up" surgery is necessary for a small number of patients. The need for a touch up depends on the skill of the doctor, the patient's natural healing process, and the patient's desire for perfection.

Chin Augmentations and Reductions

The recovery for the "alloplastic" chin implant is much less than bone advancement procedures, primarily due to the invasiveness of the procedures. Most patients can return to work the next day, but many will not return to work until after the chin bandage and support have been removed in five to seven days. With the bone advancement procedure, many have more swelling and bruising. The recovery is usually a few days to a week longer than the implant procedure.

The risks involved with both procedures include injury to the nerves that supply sensation to the lower lip and chin. Heavy bleeding in the first week is a rare problem with genioplasty. Chin implant movement and subsequent asymmetry are also a complication seen in a small percentage of patients. Infection is an even smaller complication, with more risk for the intra-oral alloplastic chin placement method.

Results

The wonderful part about recovering from nose work is that after five days, your nose generally looks normal. In most cases, no one will be able to tell that you've had anything done. People will comment that you look different — better! But they may not be sure exactly *why* until you tell them.

The majority of patients are delighted with the results of a skillfully done rhinoplasty. While it doesn't happen to everyone, sometimes the new nose promotes a transformation in the patient's self-confidence. Some individuals who have been uncomfortable with their noses for years feel as though they have been "set free." A badly formed nose can make a false statement about a person. It can make you appear mean or angry. When you can suddenly see yourself looking softer and happier, your attitude can't help but improve.

Chin implants can produce a very impressive effect for very little recovery time or expense. The implant must be matched carefully to the face or somewhat unnatural results can occur. But an implant can be easily removed if the effect is unsatisfactory. Genioplasty is a bigger deal, with a rougher recovery. Results in a skilled surgeon's hands are sometimes even better, however.

℞ Patient Stories ℘

John, age 37

I had a very fat neck and a chin that wasn't very big. When the doctor did my liposuction and put in a chin implant, I had a whole new face without any other surgery. It was a pretty easy recovery. I look a lot stronger.

Ellen, age 26

I had a classic ethnic nose, and it became a real problem when I decided in my teens that I wanted to be a model. Every photograph of me looked just terrible! I dreamed about getting my nose done for years, and when I finally got old enough, I had it done. Now I look great — I don't have this big thing in the middle of my face, and I think I look just beautiful. I've also started getting some modeling work, though there's no way to know for sure if the new nose has anything to do with it. I bet that it does.

Mark, age 35

I've had allergies and sinus problems since I was a kid. I could never breathe properly. A few years ago I had rhinoplasty to correct the medical condition that caused this, and life has been completely different ever since. While the doctor was working on my nose, he also shaved off a bit of extra bone here and there to reshape the whole thing. I love the new look, and I love being able to breathe comfortably for the first time in my life.

Office Photo Album
A Pictorial of My Work

About our photographs: we are not professional photographers, and some of the lighting, distances, and composition may not be perfectly identical in the "before" and "after" photos.

For liposuction photos, the distance from the person to the camera is critical. The patients in our liposuction photos are the *same distance* from the camera in the "before" and "after" photographs. If you are judging a doctor's work, watch for this. If the "after" photo is taken too far away, a deceptive "photographic reduction" has been done.

While these results are representative of our work, not everyone will get results like these. All work was performed by Dr. Yoho except for his personal liposuction. Our original photographs are available for our patients to examine.

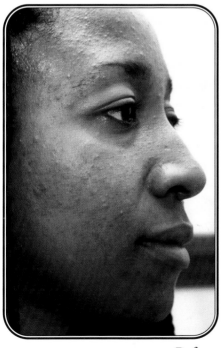
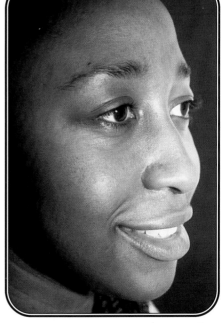

Before   After

This patient used Accutane and creams to obtain this result.
We felt that her self-image was considerably improved!

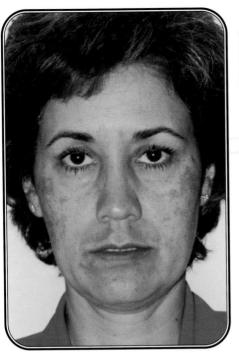 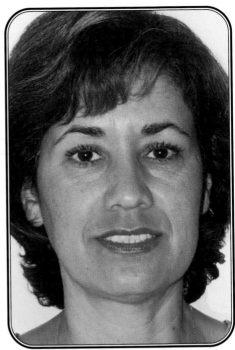

Before   After 6 weeks

Cream treatments only. Age 45 years.

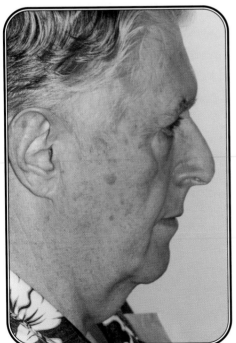 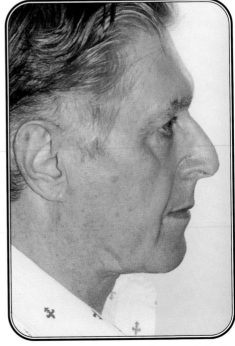

Before   After 11 Weeks

Chin and jowl liposuction. (good skin shrinkage). Age 67 years.

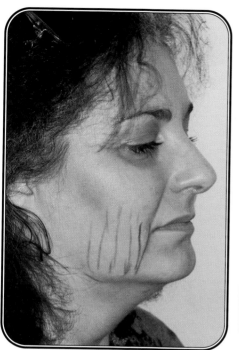
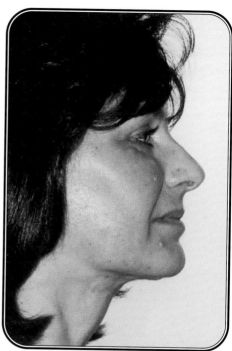

Before   After 14 Weeks

Chin and jowl liposuction (note pre-procedure marks). Age 47 years.

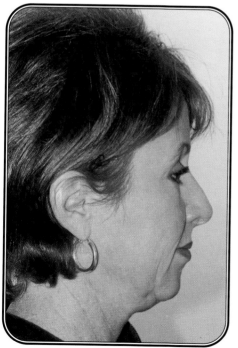
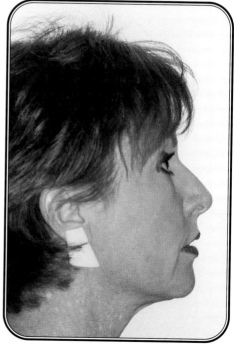

Before   After

Neck liposuction and chin implant.

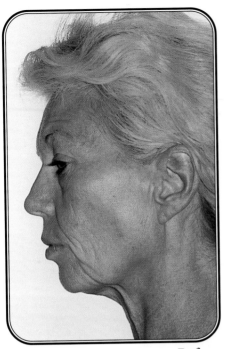
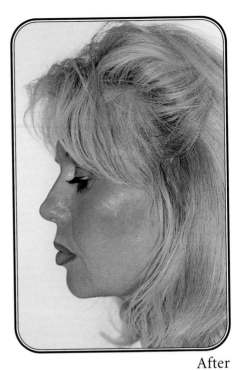

Before   After

Facial fat and laser after four months. Patient wearing make-up in
"after" photo. Notice how chin skin shrank also. (No face-lift.)

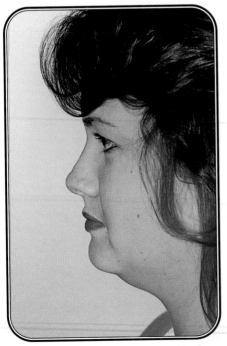
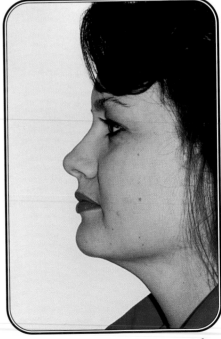

Before   After

Chin liposuction only.

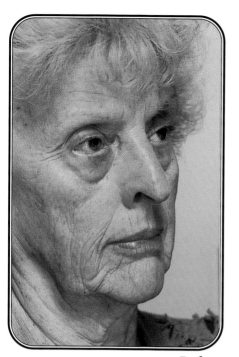
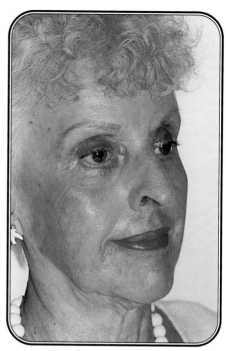

Before   After

Laser peel, lower & upper blepharoplasty, chin and jowl liposuction.
Result at two months. A little make-up in the "after" picture.

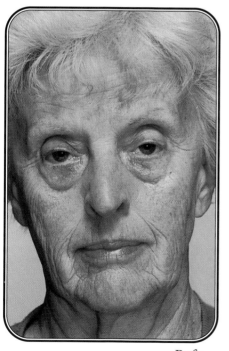
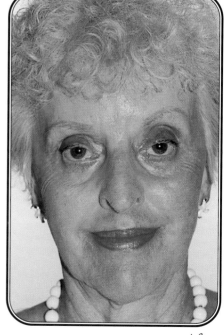

Before   After

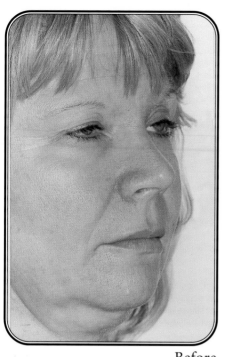
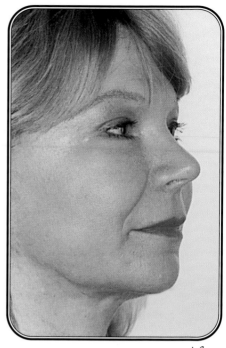

Before   After

Chin liposuction and fat transplant to lower eye area.
Make-up in the "after" picture.

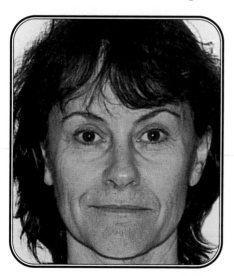
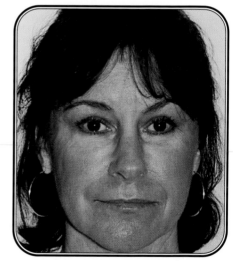

Before   After

Lines are quite pronouced   After treatment, noticeable softness

Laser resurfacing, upper blepharoplasty, facial fat transplant.

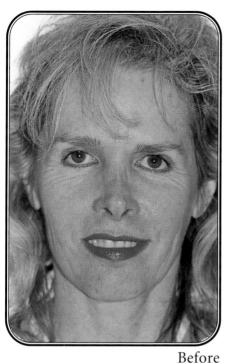

Before
"Before" facial fat and
laser resurfacing.

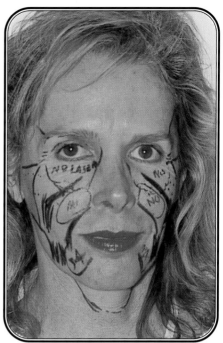

Before
Marks used to guide the doctor
where to put the fat.

**The process of
facial rejuvenation.**

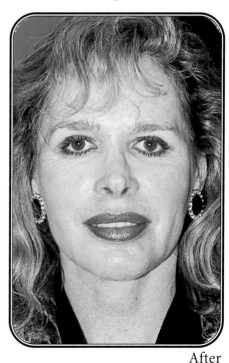

After
After facial fat and laser
resurfacing. With make-up.

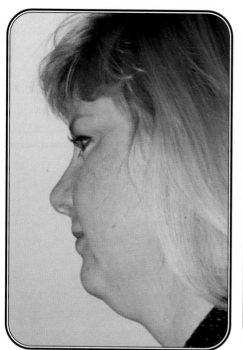
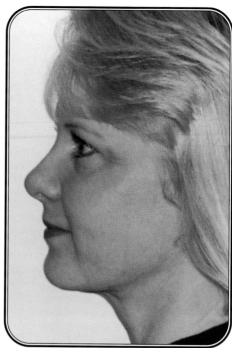

Before   After 19 weeks

Chin and jowl liposuction. Notice impressive skin shrinkage. Age 38 years.

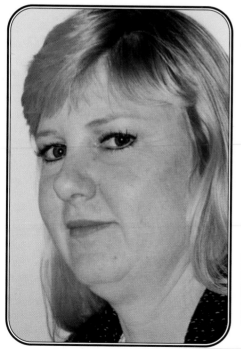
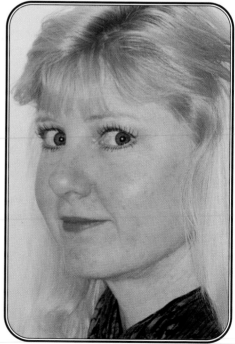

Before   After

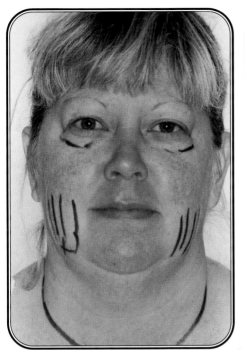 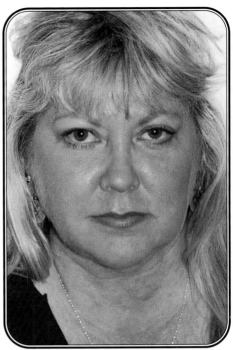

Before   After 7 weeks
Lower blepharoplasty and chin and jowl liposuction.
Age 48 years. Notice pre-procedure marks.

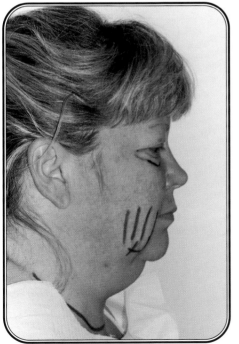 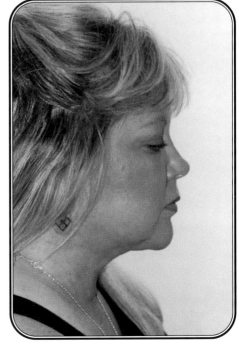

Before   After

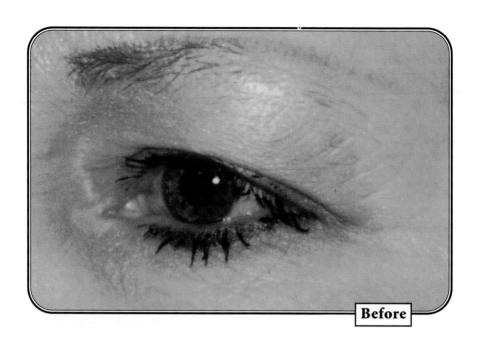

Before

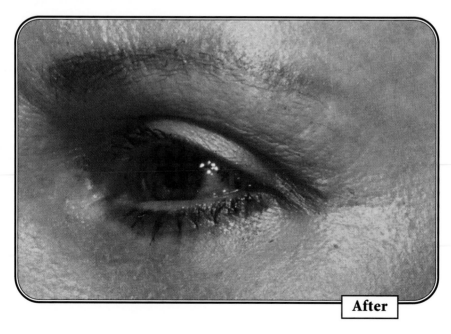

After

Repair of upper eyelids alone often makes a big difference.

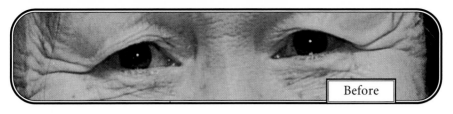

Upper blepharoplasty only for an Asian makes
her look much more alert. She's 70 years old.

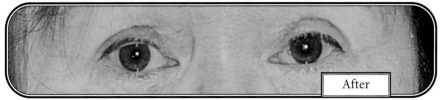

Laser resurfacing and fat transfer to lips, 52 years old.

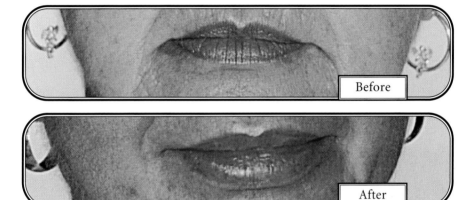

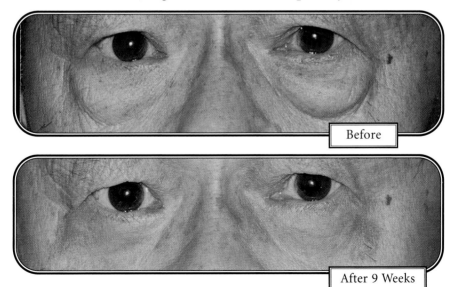

Laser blepharoplasty and lower eyelid skin resurfacing only.
(Needs upper blepharoplasty.) 73 years old.

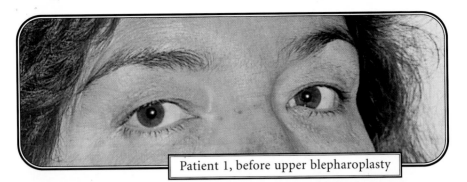

Patient 1, before upper blepharoplasty

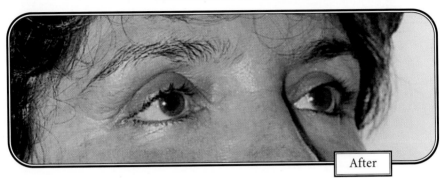

After

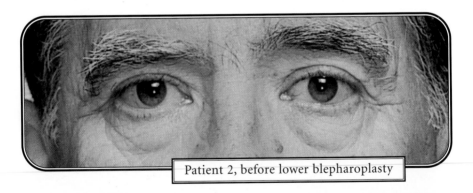

Patient 2, before lower blepharoplasty

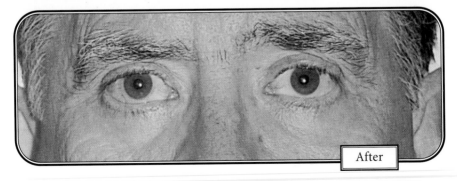

After

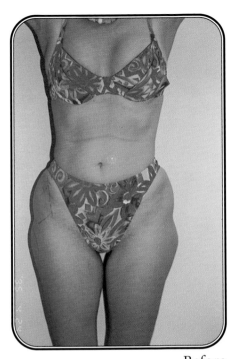 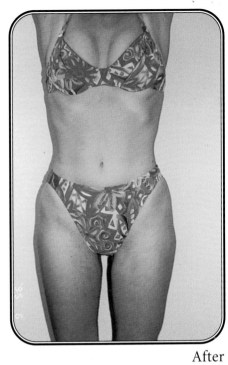

Before   After

Body liposuction.

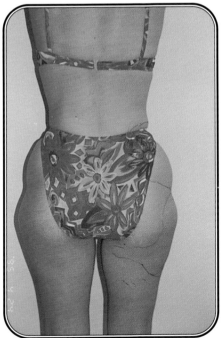 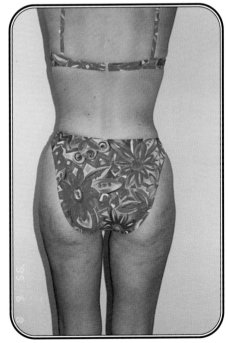

Before   After

Notice pre-surgical marks on the right hip.

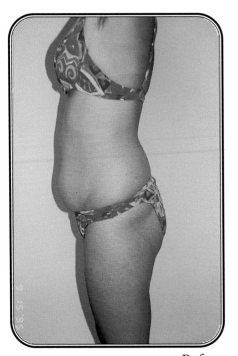 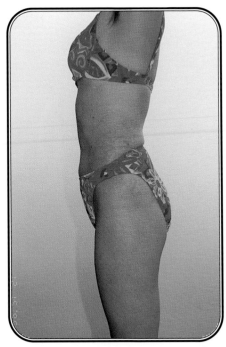

Before   After

Liposuction.

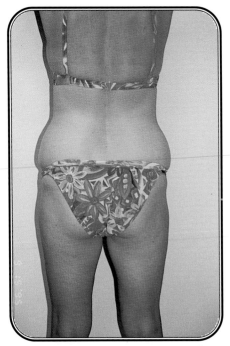 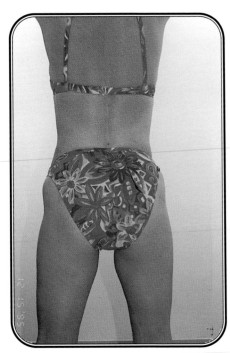

Before   After

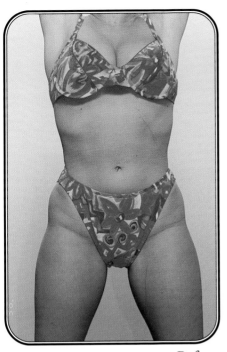

Before

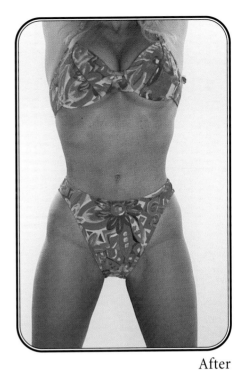

After

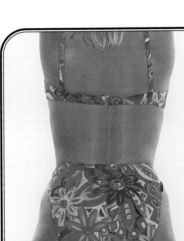

Before

After

Notice pre-liposuction markings on the left and
the improvement in skin texture on the right.

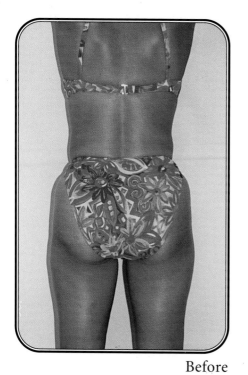 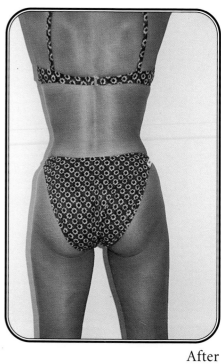

Before   After

This woman found a job as a swimsuit model after liposuction.

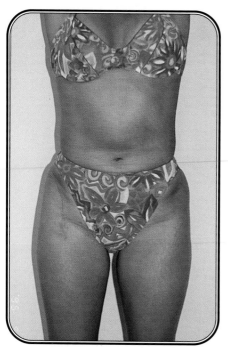 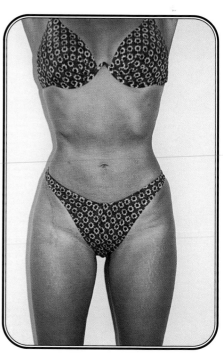

Before   After

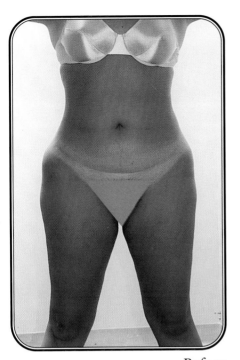 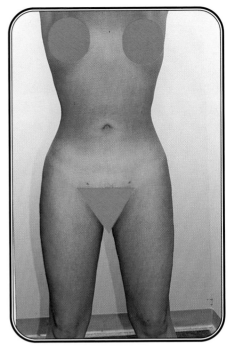

Before   After

Liposuction with a 20 pound weight loss that followed. (Patient A)

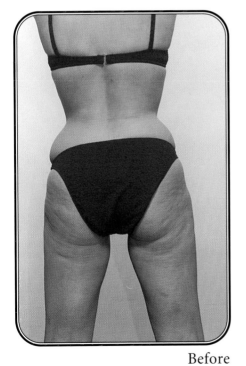 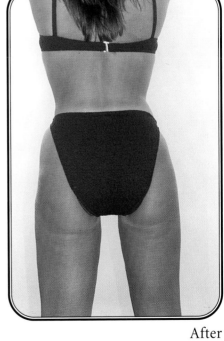

Before   After

Liposuction. (Patient B)

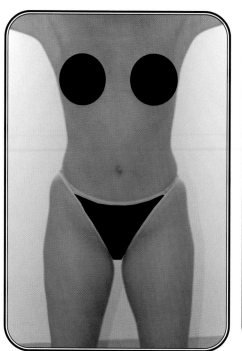
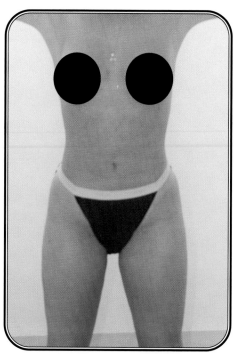

Before   After 6 Weeks

Leg and torso liposuction. 32 years old.

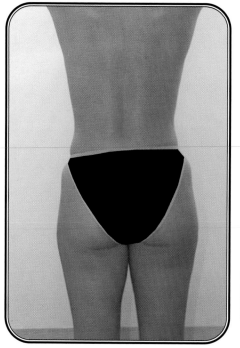
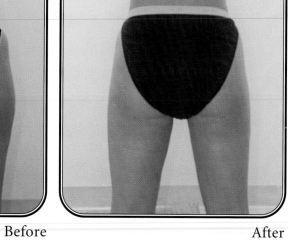

Before   After

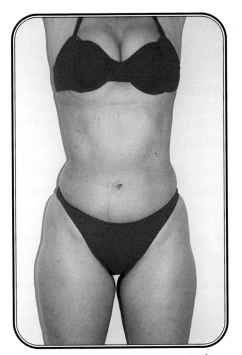
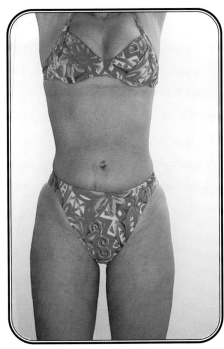

Before   After

Liposuction.

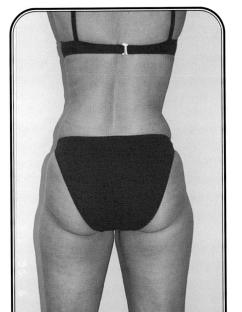
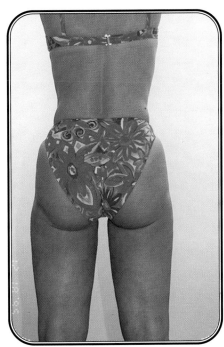

Before   After

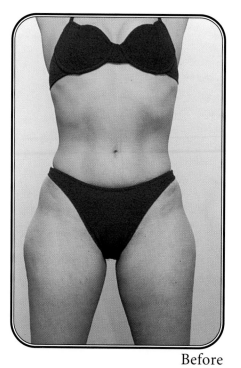
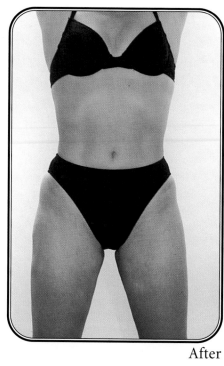

Before   After

Smaller leg cases, liposuction.

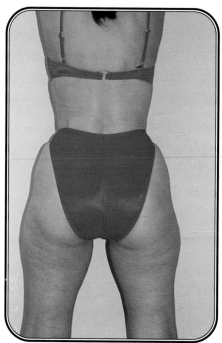
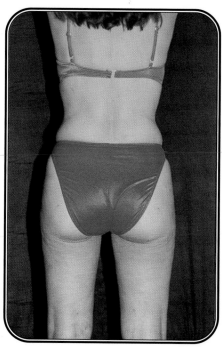

Before   After

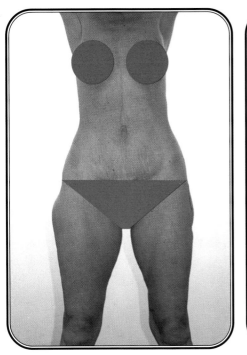 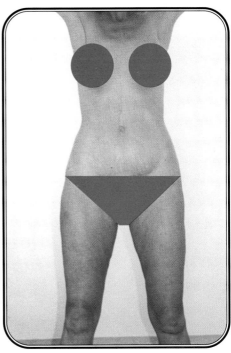

Before   After 6 weeks

Hip, inner and outer thigh and knee liposuction. 51 years old.

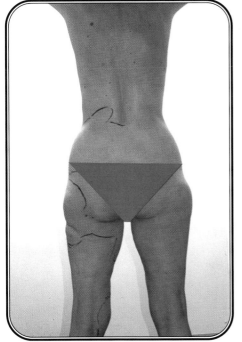 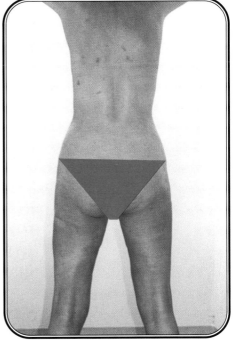

Before   After

Notice pre-procedure marking lines on before photo.

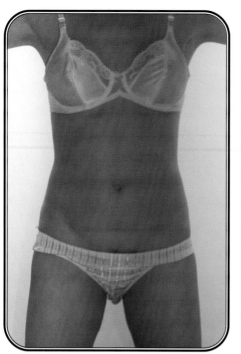
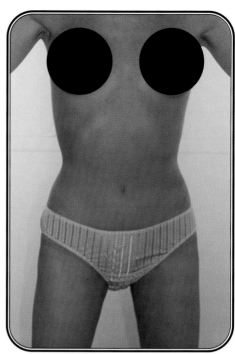

Before   After

Patient desired thinner waist. 36 years old.

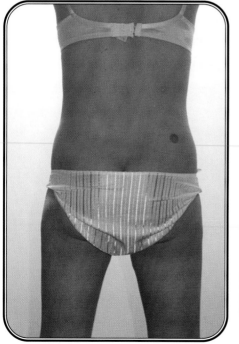
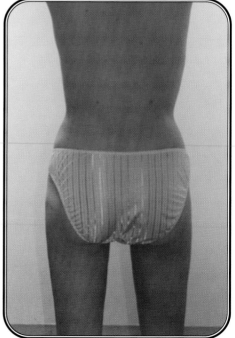

Before   After

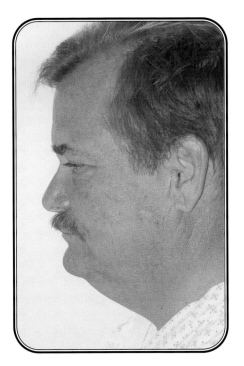 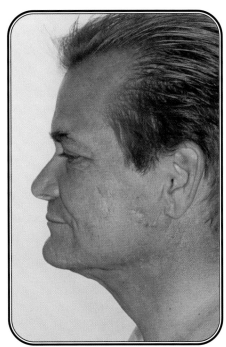

Before   After

Chin liposuction only.

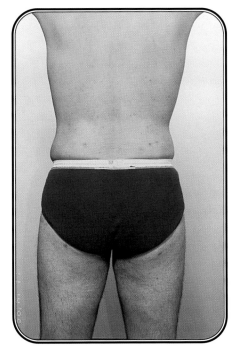 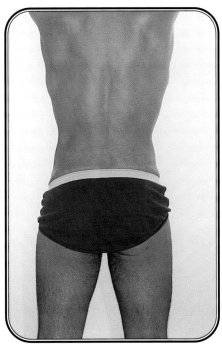

Before   After

Torso liposuction.

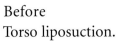

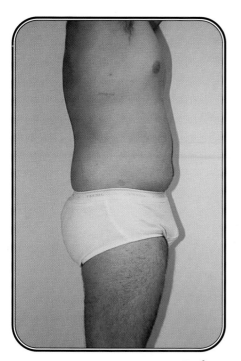 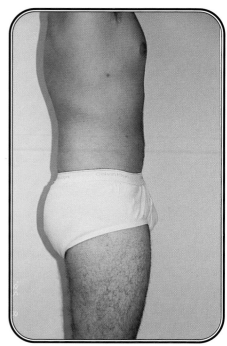

Before   After

Torso liposuction.

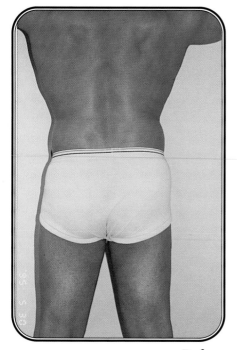 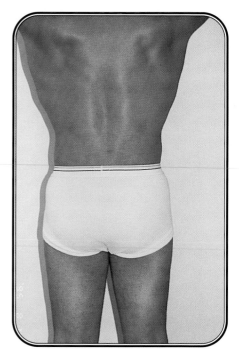

Before   After

"Love handle" liposuction.

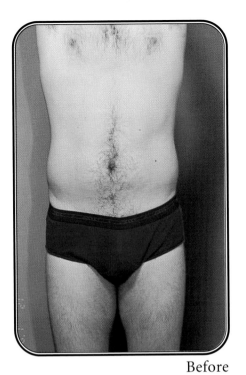
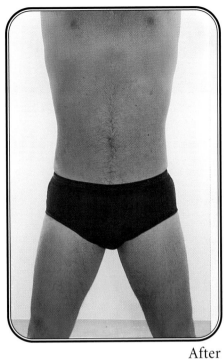

Before   After

Male cases of torso liposuction.

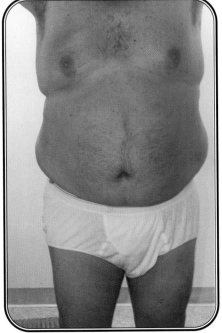
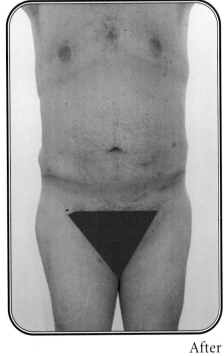

Before   After

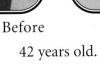

42 years old.

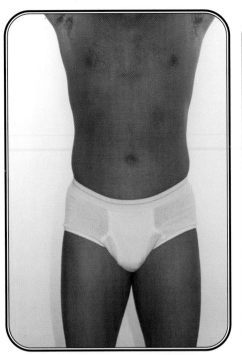 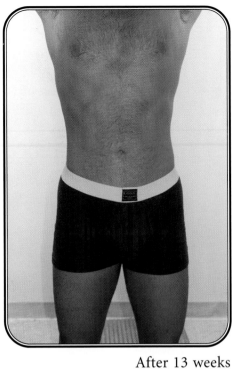

Before   After 13 weeks

Torso liposuction. Age 28 years.

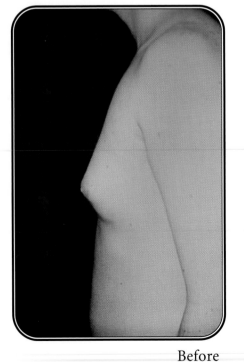 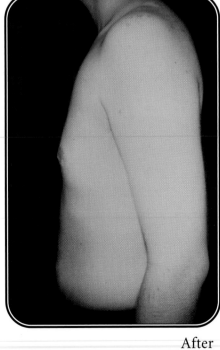

Before   After

Liposuction treatment of 22 year old male breast patient.
This breast tissue is called "gynecomastia".

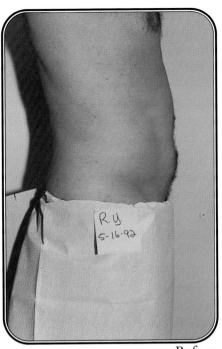
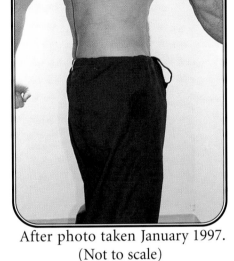

Before

After photo taken January 1997.
(Not to scale)

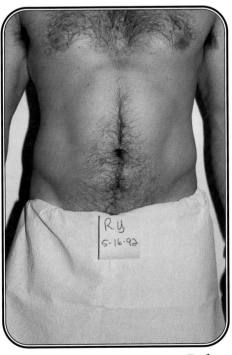
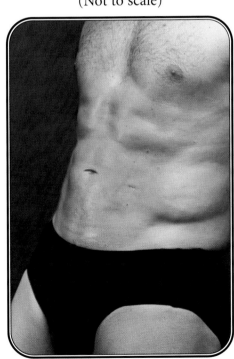

Before

After photo taken 7-09-98

Dr. Yoho had two liposuction procedures and did some bodybuilding. No, he did not liposuction himself! The small scar to the left of the doctor's navel is from an endoscopic hernia repair, not from liposuction.

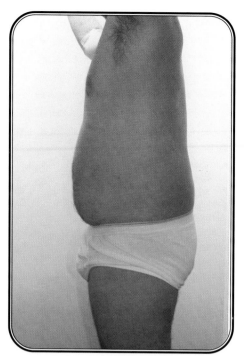 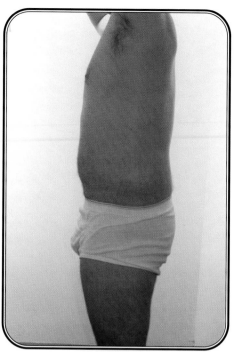

Before After

Torso liposuction.

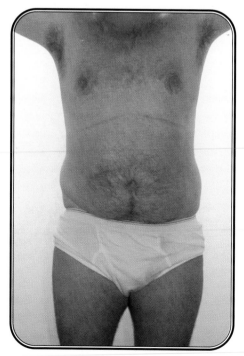 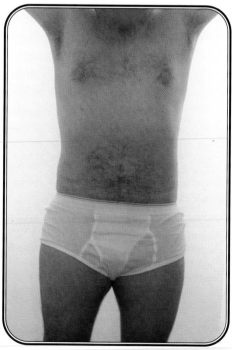

Before After

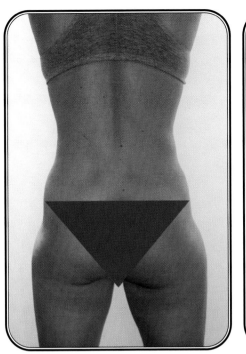 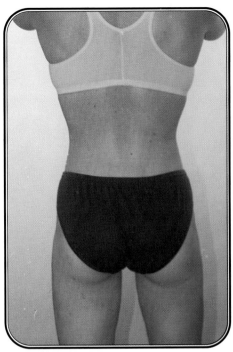

Before   After 21 Weeks

Outer and inner thigh and hip liposuction for an athletic women. 27 years old.

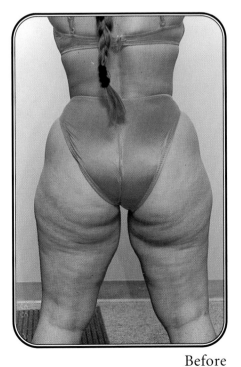 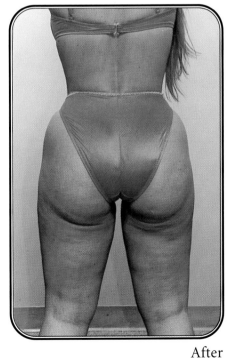

Before   After

Note that the area under the buttocks was sculptured in this case.

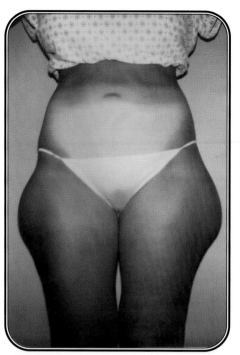
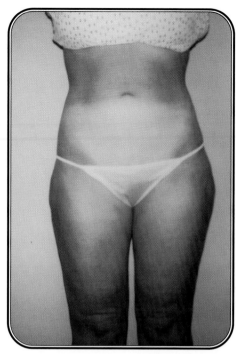

Before   After 9 Weeks

Saddlebag liposuction only. This woman ran the
L.A. Marathon both before and after her procedure.

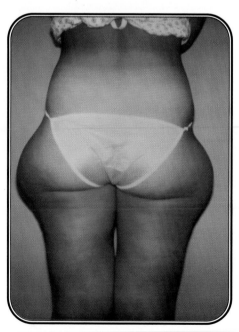
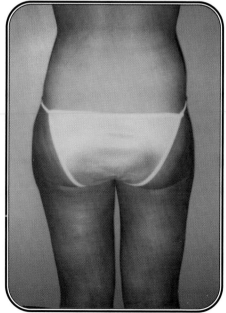

Before   After

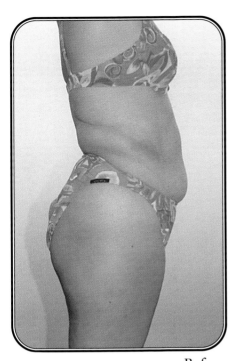
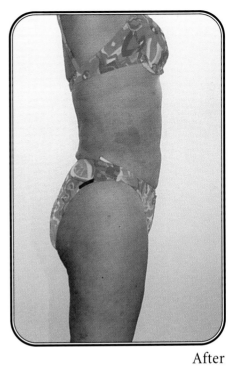

Before   After

Liposuction. (Patient A)

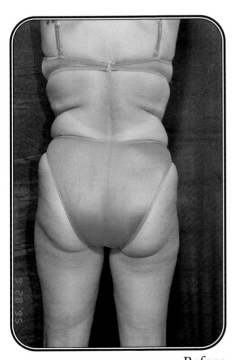
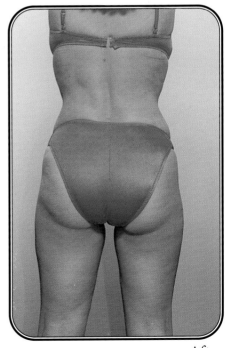

Before   After

Liposuction. (Patient B)

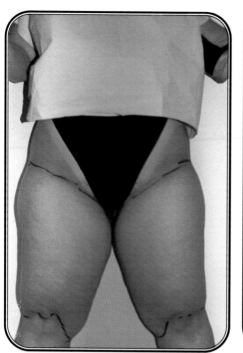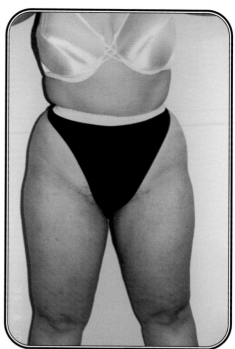

Before   After

Total leg liposuction. Note pre-procedure marks.

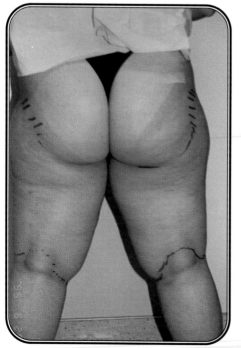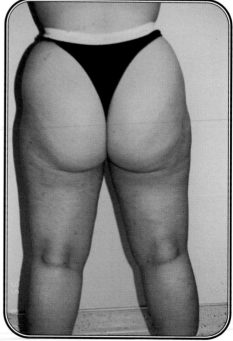

Before   After

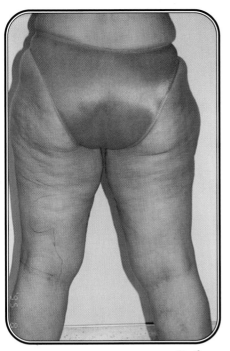 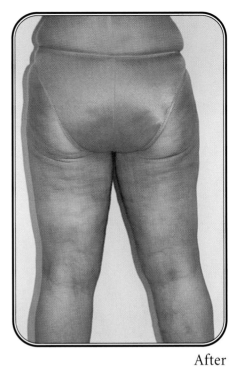

Before   After

Total leg liposuction. This must be done
very carefully with a very small cannula.

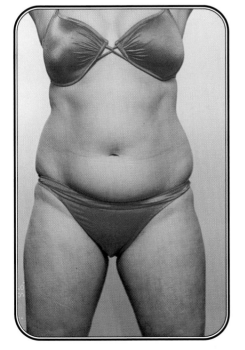 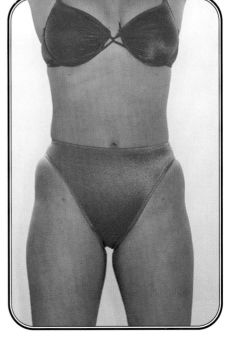

Before   After

Torso liposuction.

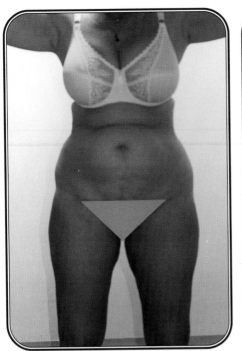
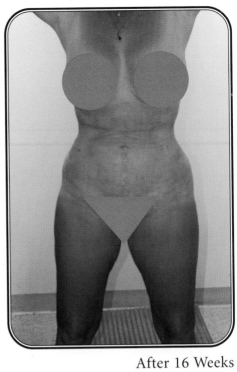

Before   After 16 Weeks

Torso liposuction. Age 61 years.

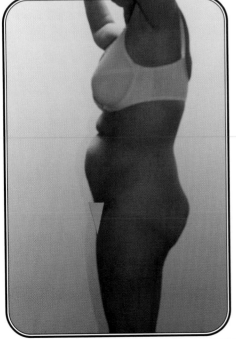
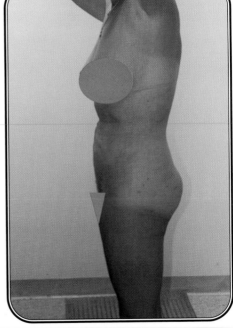

Before   After

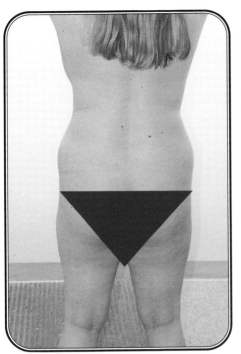
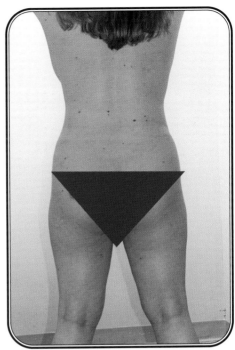

Before   After

Torso liposuction.

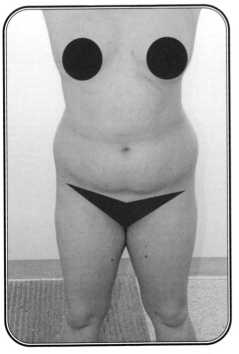
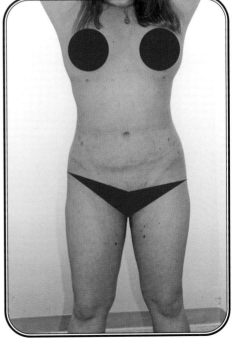

Before   After

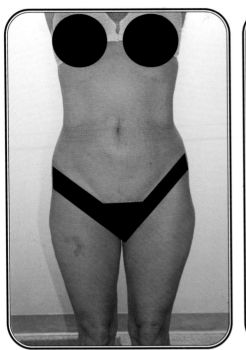 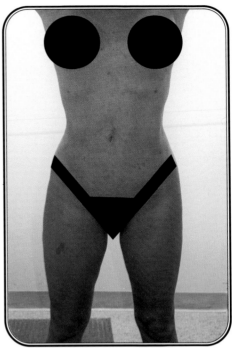

Before   After 4 1/2 months

Body liposuction. 59 years old.

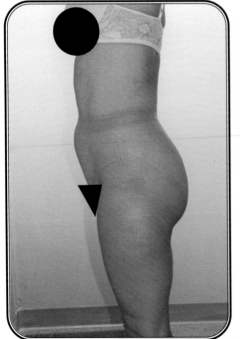 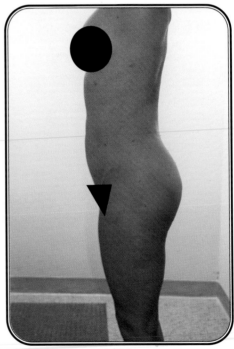

Before   After

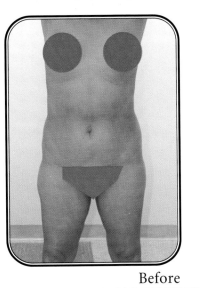

Torso and leg
liposuction.
51 years old.

Before · After

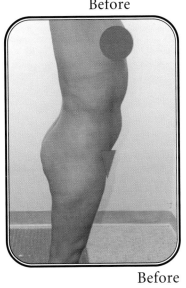

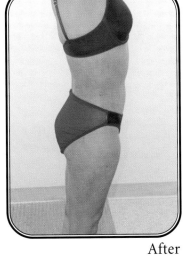

Before · After

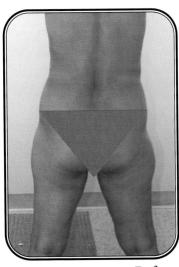

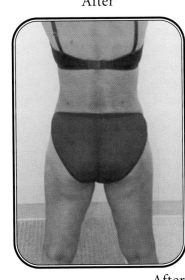

Before · After

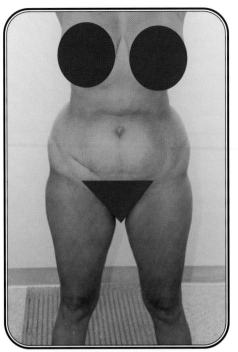
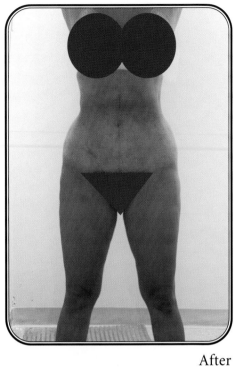

Before   After

Torso and leg liposuction. 45 years old.

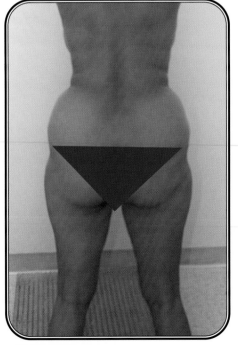
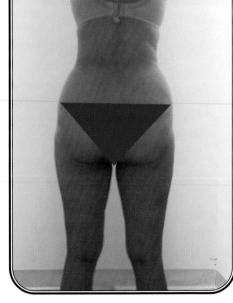

Before   After

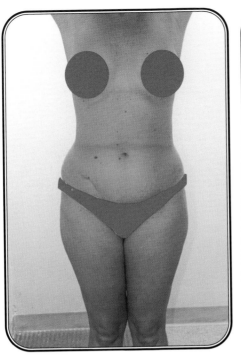 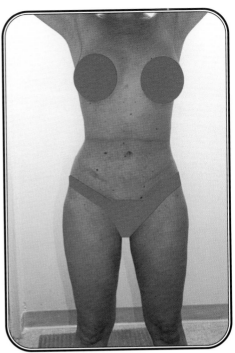

Before   After

Leg and torso liposuction. Note improvement in sunken appendectomy
scar on the patient's lower right abdomen. 34 years old. (Patient A)

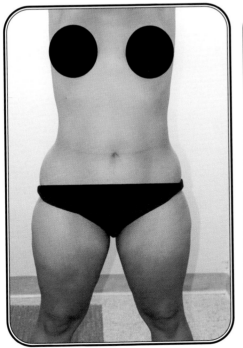 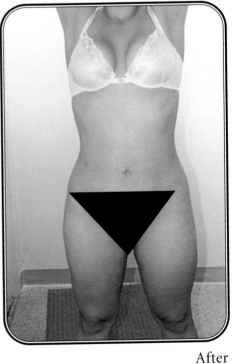

Before   After

Leg and torso liposuction. 25 years old. (Patient B)

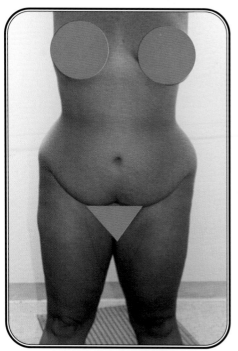 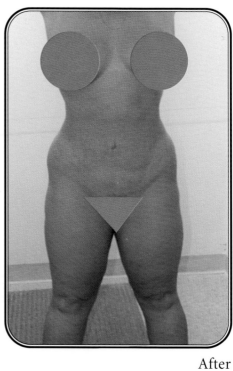

Before   After

Note skin shrinkage on the abdomen and disappearance
of the overhang after liposuction. 34 years old.

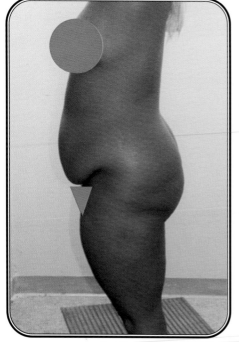 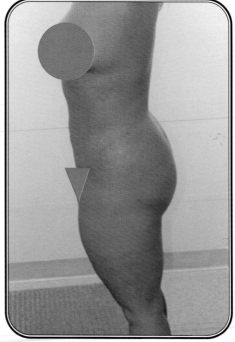

Before   After

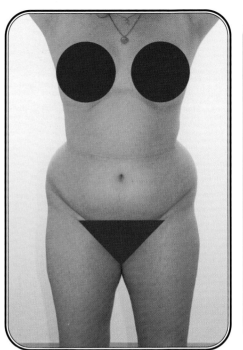 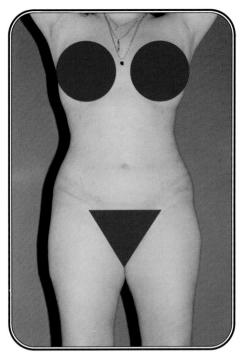

Before   After 1 month

Body liposuction. 30 years old.

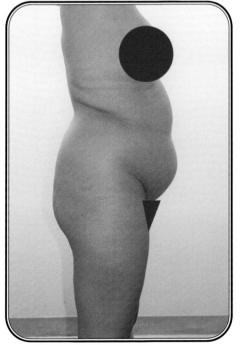 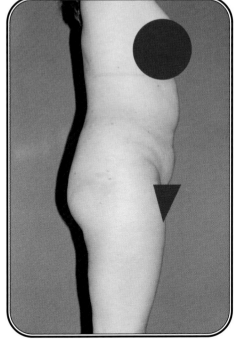

Before   After

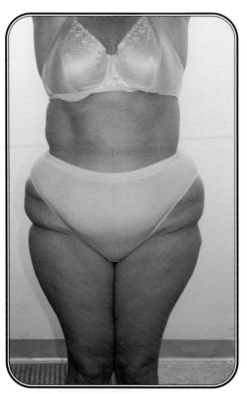

Patient A.
31 years old.
Front view.

Before

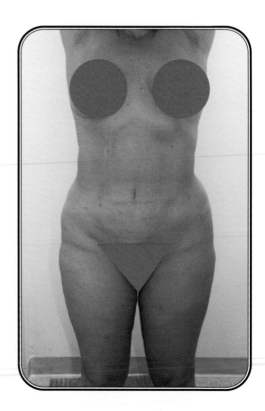

After 2 procedures.

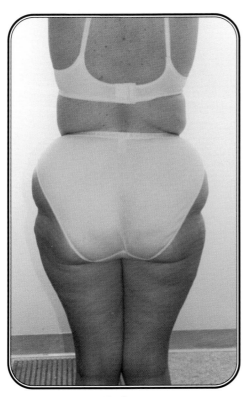

Patient A.
31 years old.
Back view.

Before

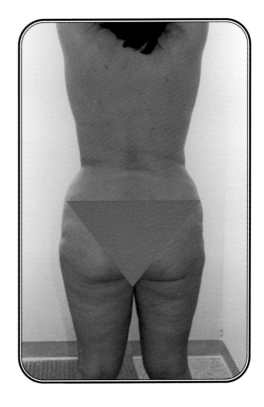

After 2 procedures.

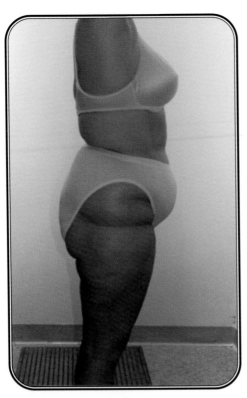

Before

Patient A.
31 years old.
Side view.

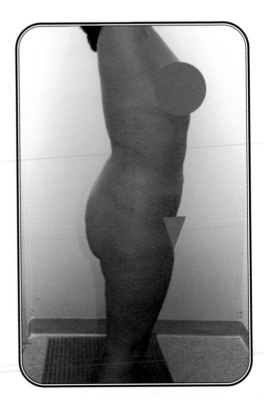

After 2 procedures.

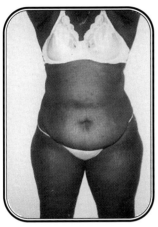 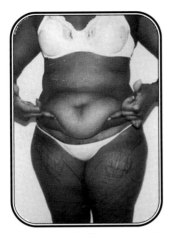 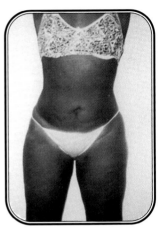

Before, view 1.	Before, view 2.	After

The "No Scalpel Tummy Tuck." Notice the amount of skin shrinkage that occurs after just a liposuction without any skin being cut out surgically.

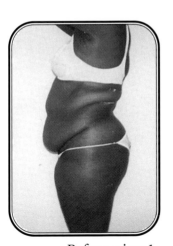 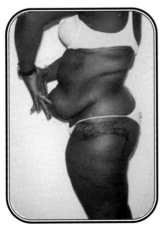 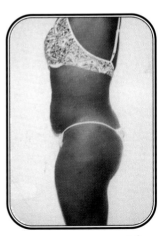

Before, view 1.	Before, view 2.	After

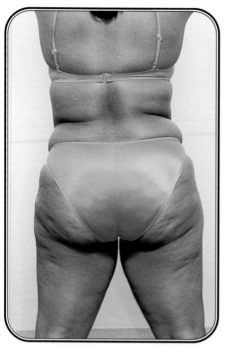 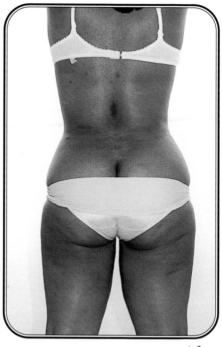

Before   After

Torso liposuction.

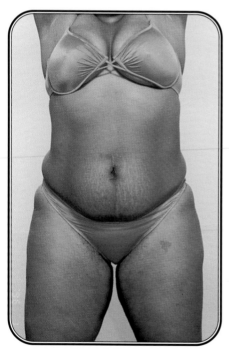 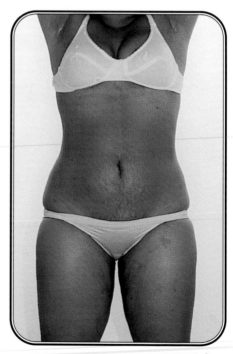

Before   After

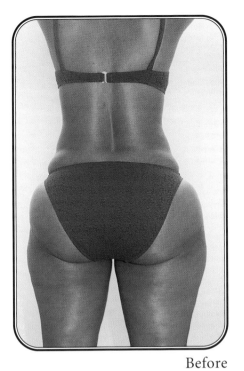 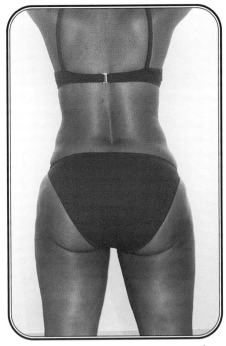

Before   After

Big leg liposuction case.

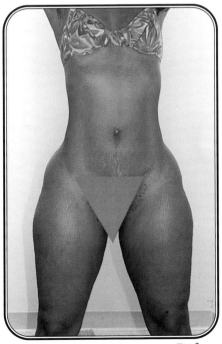 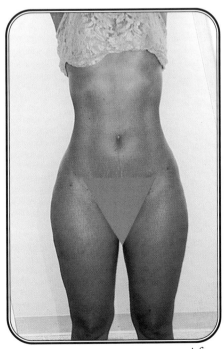

Before   After

"Double hump" liposuction case.

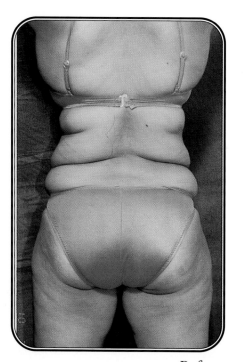
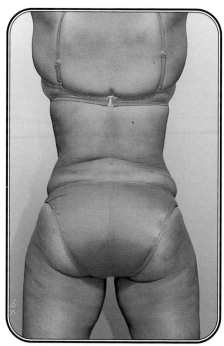

Before

After

Body liposuction. Notice dramatic skin shrinkage.

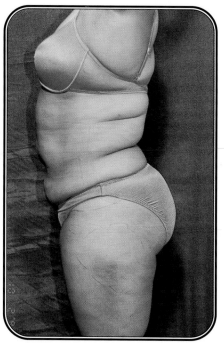
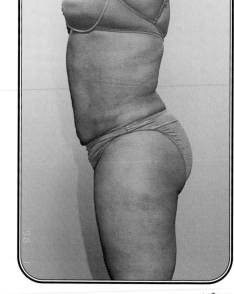

Before

After

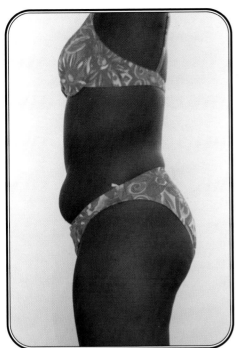 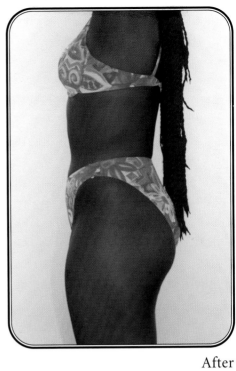

Before   After

Abdomen and hip liposuction. 27 years old.

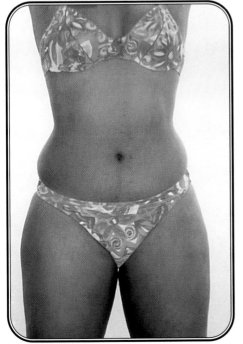 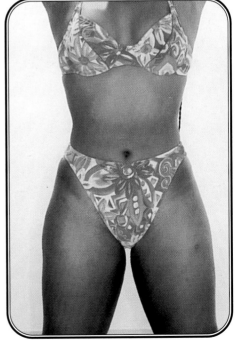

Before   After

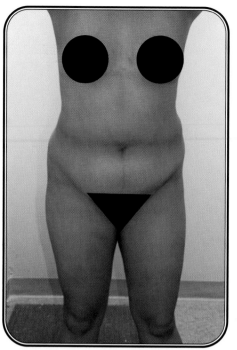
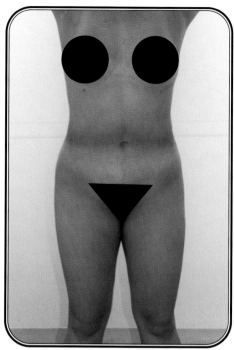

Before

After 8 Weeks

Torso liposuction only. 23 years old.

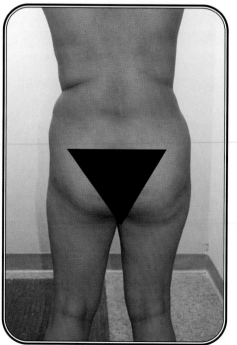
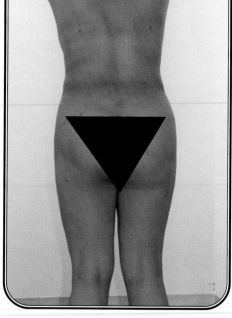

Before

After 8 Weeks

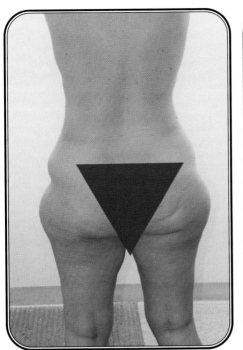
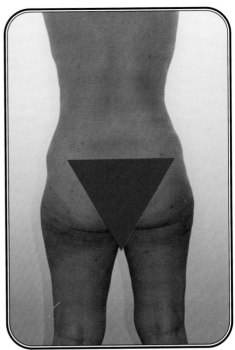

Before · After 5 weeks

Lower body liposuction. 43 years old.

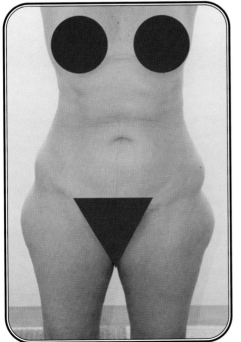
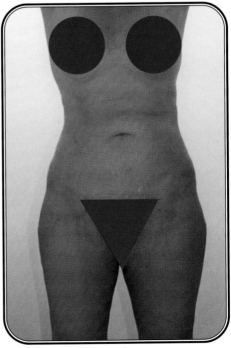

Before · After 5 weeks

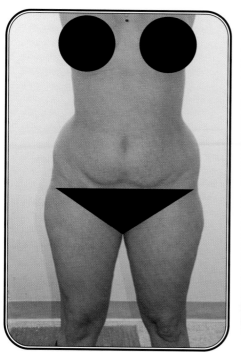 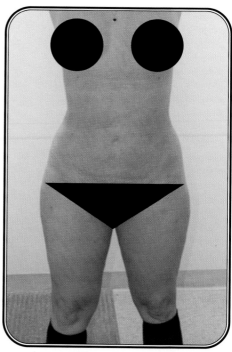

Before   After 1 month

Torso liposuction. 45 years old. (Patient A)

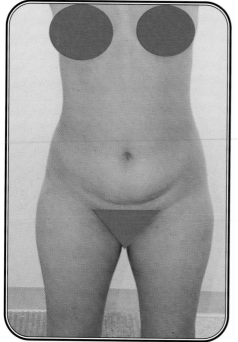 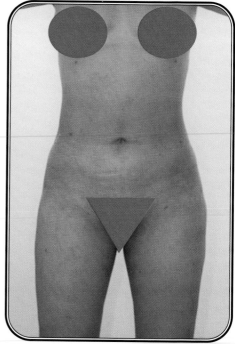

Before   After 13 weeks

Torso liposuction. 30 years old. (Patient B)

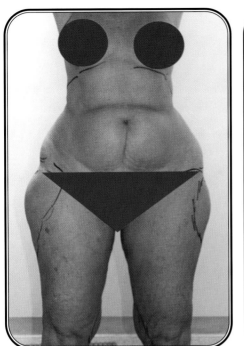 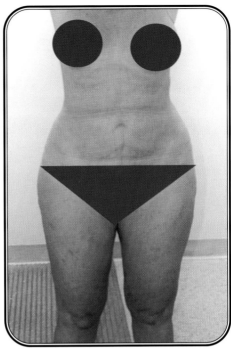

Before · After

Torso and leg liposuction. 62 years old.

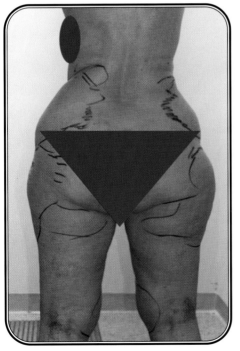 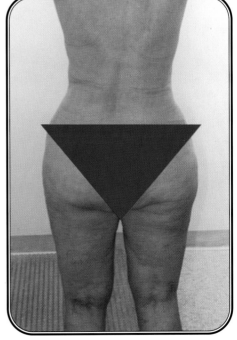

Before · After

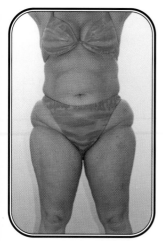
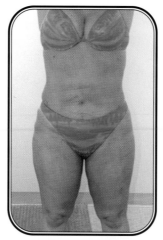

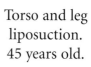
Torso and leg liposuction. 45 years old.

Before

After 5 weeks.

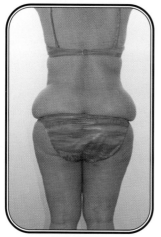
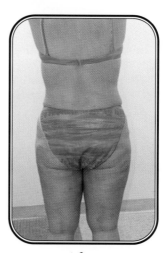

Before

After

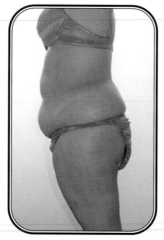
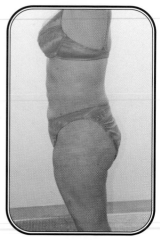

Before

After

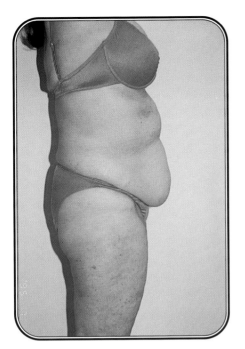 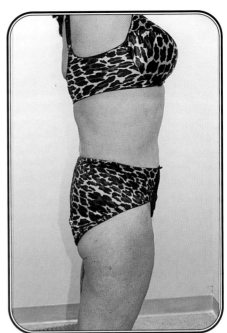

Before   After

Liposuction of body and legs plus cellulite treatment of legs.

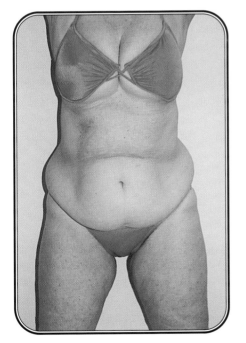 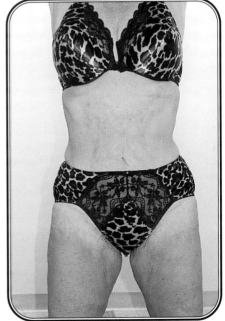

Before   After

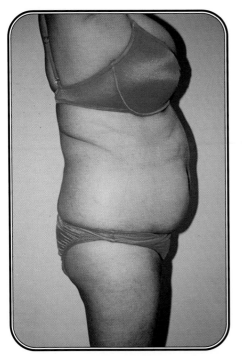
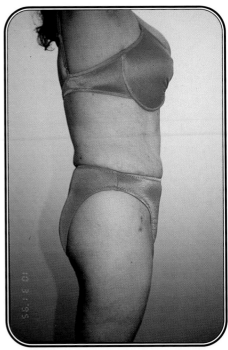

Before   After

Body liposuction.

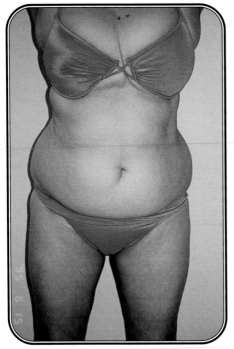
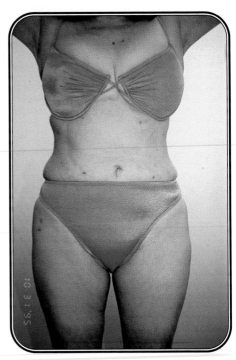

Before   4 1/2 months after.

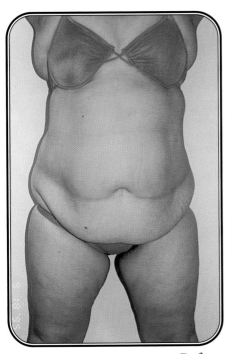
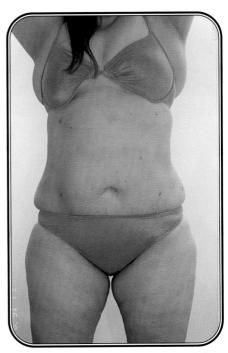

Before   After

The "No Scalpel Tummy Tuck."
Notice how the skin shrinks without any cutting or scars.
These are two different people.

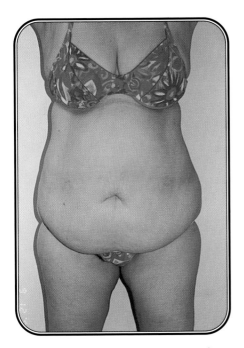
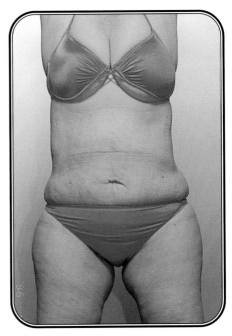

Before   After

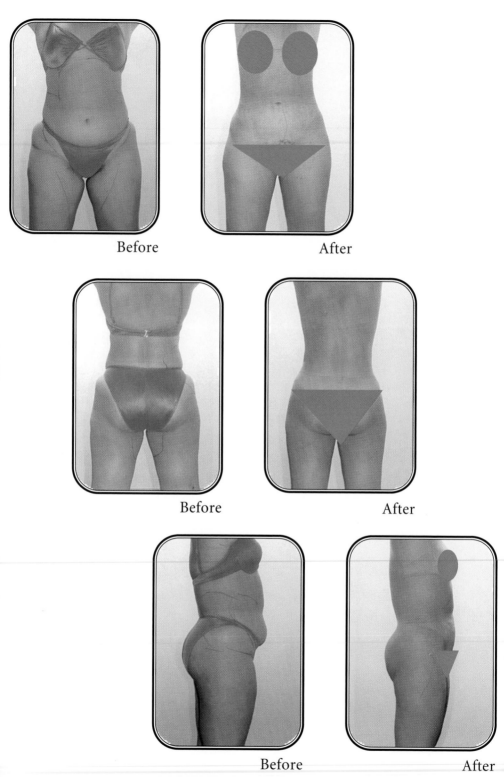

Before

After

Before

After

Before

After

Liposuction of legs and torso and a ten pound weight loss.

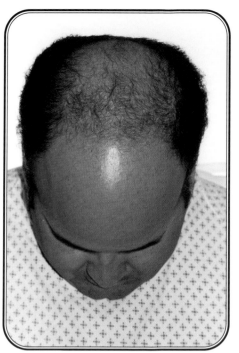
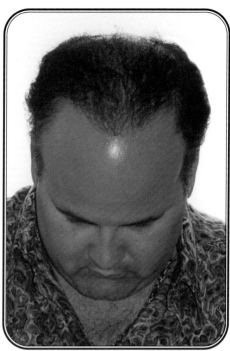

Before   After

1,000 3-hair grafts in one day.

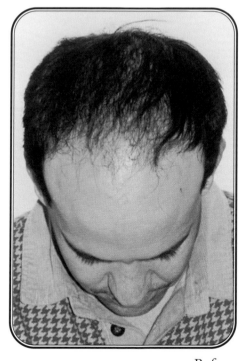
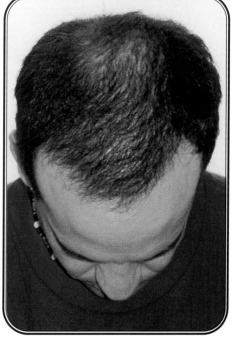

Before   After

1200 3-hair grafts in one day.

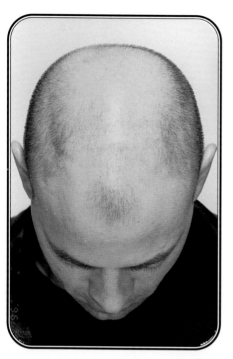
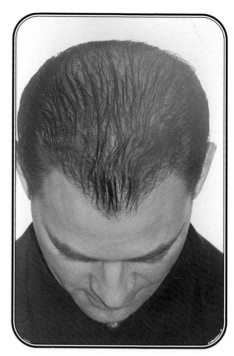

Before   After

Hair Transplant, 2,000 grafts. Note that this patient
had some hair before transplants were performed.

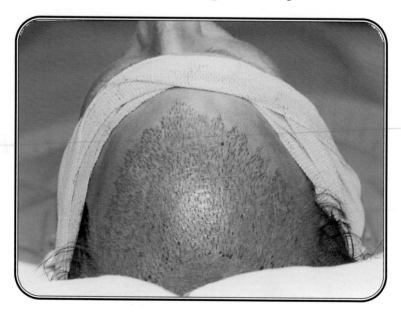

What 1,000 hair transplant grafts look like just after placement.

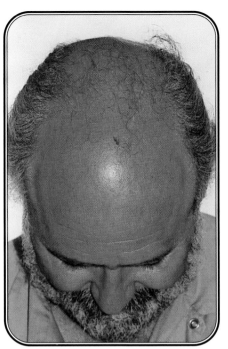 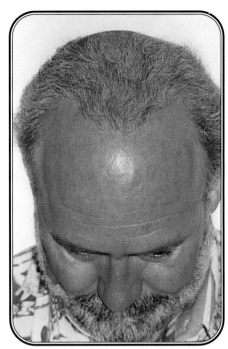

Before   After

Hair transplant: this case was only 1,200 grafts of 3 hairs each.
This took one session of 5 1/2 hours.

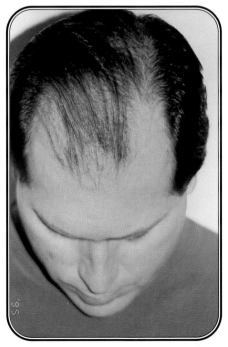 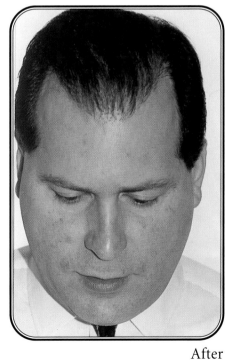

Before   After

Hair transplant, about 2,000 grafts of 3 hairs each.
Slight rotation of "After" photograph.

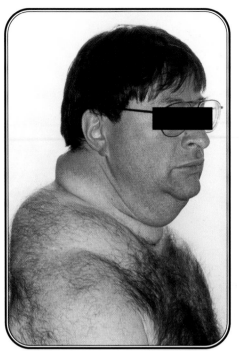
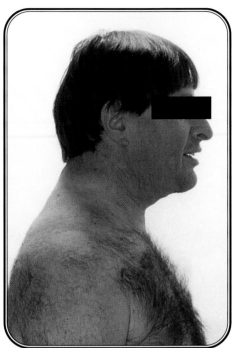

Before   After 7 Weeks

This patient has Madeline's Syndrome, or abnormal fatty tumors.
He was treated with liposuction.

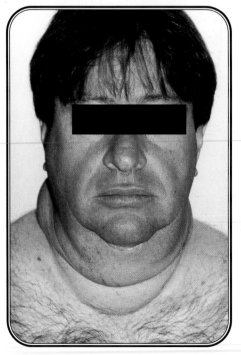
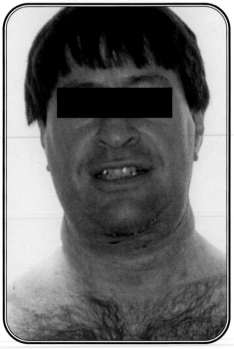

Before   After

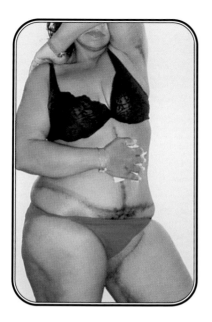

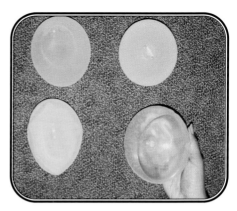

Sample breast implants for
demonstration purposes.

The patient above and the patient below had old-style "tummy tucks" (surgical reduction procedures) performed by unknown physicians. Modern liposuction can sometimes produce an excellent result in cases like these without all the scarring. Notice the distortion of the lady's hips in the photo at the lower left. This problem is called a "dog ear." The photo on the lower right was after liposuction improvement of the "dog ears."

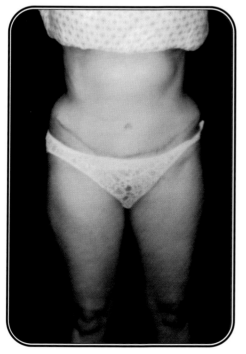

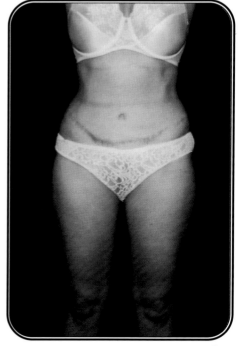

Before

After

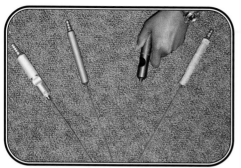

Cannulas used for liposuction.

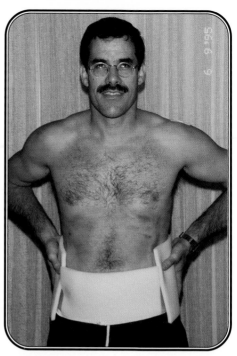

Dr. Yoho taking off his foam
5 days after his liposuction.
Notice there is some bruising.

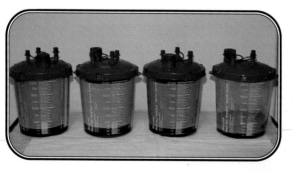

Patients always ask us, "What
does the fat look like?"
The red at the bottom is fluid
with a tiny amount of blood.

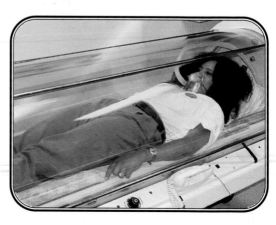

A patient inside a
hyperbaric chamber.

Fat Transplantation

❧ *For making a body part fuller, modern fat transplantation is more reliable and safer than anything else which has been developed to date.*

❧ *Fat can now be transplanted almost anywhere in the body, with good chances of long-term "take."*

❧ *When combined with laser peeling, careful fat transplants to the aging face can produce stunning, long lasting improvement.*

❧ *Swelling after the procedure is somewhat prolonged, although the hyperbaric chamber can shorten this problem considerably.*

Most of us cannot stand the sight of our own fat. We spend billions of dollars and lots of precious time trying to make it disappear. Most of us, at one time or another, have wished that we could simply remove the fat from one area of the body and "transplant" it to another. In the mid 1990s, over 50,000 people a year did just that.

Fat that has been removed from one part of the body can be injected into other parts, most commonly lips, cheeks, breasts, buttocks, face, calves, pectorals and even the penis. Historically, the medical community has known about fat transplants for over thirty years, but its popularity has soared in the last five. The procedure is extremely safe, there are almost no side effects, and it can be done in a few hours in a doctor's office. The only real problem is that the results have frequently been unpredictable, because until recently, there's been no way to anticipate how well the body will retain the newly placed fat. In some experiments, fat that's been chemically labeled has been injected and then checked years later, revealing itself to be perfectly intact. But retention has varied widely from one patient to the next and from one doctor to the next, in large part because fat injection and harvesting techniques can vary. Some patients retain 100 percent, while others retain none at all. In some parts of the body, fat can simply melt off, the same way it melts off with dieting and exercise.

Only in the past few years have we had any methods to standardize fat transfer. Sydney Coleman, a physician from New York City, has been doing brilliant work with this problem since the mid 1980s. He has pioneered fat transplanting techniques that result in remarkable long-term fat retention, and his photographs show just how well his techniques work, with excellent results maintained over the years. His special instruments and low suction treat the harvested fat very gently. Additionally, the fat is carefully spread out into the transplanted area, producing better nutritional support for the injected material and more even results. The method is very time consuming, but the results make it worthwhile. We use these new tools and techniques in our surgical center and have had beautiful results.

Where and Why to Transplant Fat

People seek fat transplants for a variety of reasons. For example, a good candidate for transplantation of fat into the breasts might be a post-nursing woman who's lost some volume and whose skin is slightly sagging, but not enough for more serious breast surgery such as mastopexy or breast implants. A fat transplant can fill the breast and sometimes restore or improve its original shape. In many cases, this may be preferable to artificial implants. Of course, fat doesn't have the potential to produce the extra-large breasts some women want.

When fat is injected into breasts, the interior structure of the breast changes slightly. "Calcification" may occur, which shows up on a mammogram. This happens whenever soft tissue is manipulated and can also happen from minor bruising. Calcification can also occur with breast cancer, so there is some concern about confusing fat transfer with cancer when a doctor looks at a mammogram. However, physicians who specialize in reading X rays feel that the mammogram changes which show up with fat implants or injury are generally quite different from those that occur with cancer (cancer calcifications have a distinct "stellate" or star shape). Additionally, there is no known risk of fat injection (or breast implants for that matter) triggering or stimulating cancer in breasts.

Lips and cheeks are also popular sites for fat transplantation, for everyone from movie stars to older people who just want healthy, fuller-looking lips. As we age, the face tends to lose its fullness. The fat under the skin just shrinks away, leaving a hollow, skeletal look. Have you looked at Harrison Ford in the old Star Wars movies recently? These were filmed in the 1970s, when Ford was in his early thirties. He was an attractive younger man, with heavy lips and "baby cheeks." We're all familiar with how he looks now, a more craggy character with a slight tendency towards "jowls" (loose skin in the area of the jaw near the lips). This is a normal maturation, with loss of facial fat, particularly around the mouth. His skin texture has aged, but more importantly, the fat "foundation" has gone away to some extent.

This process affects both men and women, and more quickly in light skinned persons. But we can now correct it by adding fat taken from other parts of the body. With careful "reverse sculpting" we can re-create the high cheek bones, heavy lips and full foreheads of youth. We can now add as much as eight ounces of fat to the whole face, smoothing the contours and thickening sagging areas. While some of the fat will melt away, we feel that what is seen at two to three months will stay for years.

An older, traditional approach was for doctors to put plastic "implants" in cheekbones and chins, but sometimes as the patients aged and the fat in their faces weakened and melted away, the implanted areas would remain prominent, and the whole face would look out of balance. A fat transplant generally produces smoother, more even results. "Jowling," or loose skin at the sides of the mouth, can be pulled up and corrected somewhat by fat transfer to the rest of the face. We ask our older patients to bring in photos of themselves taken when they were in their 20s or 30s, so we can see how their lips, cheeks, foreheads and eyes appeared when their faces were younger. We try to match that.

Men, particularly body builders, sometimes want to increase the size of the pectoral or calf muscles. Fat transplants can help. This procedure is remarkably successful, because Dr. Coleman has found that *fat sticks inside muscle quite well*. Because muscle has more blood supply than fat, the injected fat actually has a better life support system in muscle. The same is generally true for fat transplanted into the buttocks. However, buttocks require very large amounts of injected fat to create the desired effect.

You've no doubt heard about penis enlargement and lengthening procedures. Lengthening is done by cutting a connecting ligament that holds the penis up to the pubic bone when erect. This causes a more horizontal "angle of dangle," adding about one-half to one inch of length. Fat can be injected under the skin all around the penis, which adds thickness. It's a simple procedure which takes about 30 minutes. The fat transplanted here can be somewhat irregular, however, and because the tip of the penis is not usually filled with fat, the shaft can end up looking thicker than the tip. For those who can accept these drawbacks (and there's a market for this, believe me) and who are very motivated toward size, the operation can be very gratifying.

How It's Done

The patient is prepared for liposuction as described in chapter 3, and fat is removed in a similar manner, but with some minor differences. Instead of using a standard liposuction cannula (the instrument for suctioning the fat), a special new cannula designed by Dr. Coleman handles the flow of fat more gently. The cannula is attached to a syringe, which the doctor uses to withdraw the fat (as opposed to regular liposuction in which the fat is pumped out vigorously by a machine). This part of the procedure — removing the fat — is called "harvesting." The idea is to process the fat with extreme care, so as not to disturb its cell structure. The more intact the fat cells are, the better they will be retained in their new location.

Because the liposuction is done with a tumescent anesthetic solution (please see chapter 15 on tumescent anesthesia), there is liquid mixed in with the harvested fat. This is separated by spinning the material in a centrifuge. We then use the "processed" fat cells for injection.

The harvested fat is next injected with Dr. Coleman's tiny, specially-designed blunt cannula. We inject tiny amounts of fat at a time into different levels, just a few drops here and there. It's a slow, tedious process, and it takes hours. The treated areas can be seen expanding as the work is done.

The quantity of fat going into each area is precisely measured. The face, for example, is naturally symmetrical, so if we put a tenth of an ounce of fat on one side, then putting a tenth of an ounce on the other side should make it come out even. We "fine tune" our work visually at the end, and attempt to compensate for any uneven qualities that existed before the procedure.

If the face is being injected with fat, we routinely do a laser peel so the skin will "shrink to fit." Please see chapter 5 for a description of the laser peeling process.

Recovery

Because fat implantation is usually done in conjunction with several other procedures (liposuction and laser peeling for example), please refer to the appropriate chapters for details on how they're done and what the recovery process is like for each one.

Most doctors apply a liposuction garment or a compression dressing to the areas of your body where the fat was removed. If you've also had a laser peel, you'll usually have the laser dressing on as well. We routinely put foam and compression on facial fat transplant areas even if there was no laser treatment. On any areas which have been lasered and fat-enhanced, your recovery will be the same as it would for a standard laser peel recovery. However, the swelling will last longer because of the fat injections.

Pain is not a big deal if a full-face dressing is used (if you have much pain, get in to see your doctor right away, because you could be having a cold sore outbreak that might cause scarring). As with any laser peel, the night and day dressing on your face can be irritating. For the first day or two, it will help to ice your face many times each day for 20 minutes, with a damp washcloth or the dressing between the skin and the ice. You may also find that the swelling (and sometimes the dressing) makes it difficult to move your mouth comfortably for the first couple of days. You may receive a cortisone-type medication for swelling, an anti-viral, and an antibiotic.

Your return to normal activity depends on which part of the body was injected. For breasts, you'll need to wear a special bra for two to three weeks which is designed to keep the breasts from moving around too much and allows the fat to settle into place. The same is true for the penis. When you leave the office, it will be wrapped and taped in an upright position and should not be moved around or manipulated for two days. For facial fat transplants, the worst swelling lasts about three weeks, after which our patients are usually very pleased. Healing of the skin after a laser procedure should take between one and two weeks, and some fat loss usually continues for up to two months.

If you're lucky enough to have access to a hyperbaric chamber (see chapter 17 for more information), your swelling will decrease much faster, and the fat retention rate may also be much better.

Results/Complications

Rarely does any serious complication or side effect occur with fat transplantation. Usually the worst that can happen is some contour irregularity or no visible difference at all. If lumpiness or asymmetry occurs, careful cortisone injections or more fat transplantation usually correct the problem. Scarring is extremely rare because of the tiny needle holes that are made, and infection is unusual (possibly because of an anti-bacterial in the lidocaine anesthetic). You may need to return to see the doctor frequently for several months to be sure everything is going well. If the patient has significant weight gain after the procedure, the face can become very fat, too.

I believe that facial laser peeling combined with fat transplantation gets a better result than a face lift in many cases.

⚮ Patient Stories ♀

Victoria, age 64

I'd been thinking about having work done on my face for the last 10 years. Early this year I had a light laser peel, and I was very unhappy with my results, because I really couldn't see any difference. I'd heard about these new techniques, so I investigated. I ended up with a lower eyelid "blepharoplasty" to remove the fat from under my eyes, and liposuction in the jowl area. I also had some fat transplanted into other parts of my face at the same time to reshape the face even more.

The liposuction was a real surprise. He took fat from my stomach, and I love the way my stomach looks now. I only had this done about two weeks ago, so it's hard to tell how my face is going to look because there's still swelling. But I can already see that my chin looks more defined, and that was my biggest problem area. I can't wait to see what each new day brings.

Marilyn, age 66

I have always been kind of thin, and as I got older, it really started to show in my face. I'd heard that fat transplanted into the face could make everything look fuller, kind of puffing out the saggy spots and filling in the wrinkles. I had it done last year, and I love the results. It looks like a lot of my wrinkles actually disappeared, and my whole face looks much younger.

Breast Implants, Reduction, and Repair

This chapter was contributed by my colleague, Dr. Mani Nambiar.

☒ *Breast reconstruction has a very high patient satisfaction rate, but has a higher complication rate than most other cosmetic surgeries. This is because with implants, a "foreign" substance is left in the body.*

☒ *Modern breast implants are salt-water–filled silicone bags. The old Silicone-filled implants are not used because of lawsuit problems, although there is no medical evidence whatsoever that they cause any harm.*

☒ *Size, shape, and where to put the incision and the implant are extremely important. The patient and the doctor make these decisions as a team.*

Just as styles of clothes, architecture and music change from decade to decade, so do styles of bodies. In the 1950's, Marilyn Monroe and Jayne Mansfield epitomized America's ideal of the perfect woman's body, with round curves and ample bosoms (dress size 12 to 14!). But if either of these actresses tried to get a role in Hollywood today, they'd have to hire a personal trainer and lose 25 pounds first.

The poster girls of the 1970s and early 1980s — like Farrah Fawcett, Cheryl Tiegs, and Heather Locklear — popularized slim bodies with small breasts. Then, when the 1980s brought us aerobics, women strived to achieve tight, muscular bodies. In the course of the 1990s, large breasts once again have become part of the picture.

Many women seek breast reconstruction because their breasts are asymmetrical, or one is less developed than the other. A woman who's had a breast removed because of cancer may also desire breast reconstruction. Some women whose breasts sag after having children, or women who are unhappy about the way gravity has pulled their breasts down with age, simply may wish to revitalize them.

Occasionally men have breast surgery, because some men have excess breast tissue. It can happen for a number of different reasons: steroid use, tumors, alcohol or drug abuse, or sometimes because excess testosterone has been converted to estrogen during adolescence. Most men who are examined and tested have no clear cause for their condition. Men who have "gynecomastia" have usually been unhappy about it for many years. When it's treated successfully with aggressive liposuction, these men are among the most grateful of all cosmetic surgery patients. But when traditional invasive surgery is performed, the scar is frequently as embarrassing as the original problem.

Preparation

Just about any woman can be a candidate for breast reconstruction, whether she's interested in enlargement, reduction, or mastopexy (the repair of sagging breasts). There are many, many aspects to consider, and a patient should spend plenty of time asking questions and getting educated about her choices. There are several options in three primary areas: enlargement or reduction size, how an implant will be placed, and the type of incision that will be used.

There are several ways to enhance breasts surgically. Traditional breast augmentation enlarges the breast with an implant filled with salt water or "saline," similar to the water that makes up 70 percent of the body. The old style liquid silicone-filled implants have been removed from the marketplace and are no longer used. Breasts can also be enlarged by fat transplantation (please read chapter 9 on fat transplantation). Fat is most appropriate for tight, relatively small breasts without much saggy skin. If the patient wants a very large size, the saline implant is the way to go.

Size and Style

When you come to the doctor's office for a consultation, he will help you choose the implant size and shape that is best for you. This is done by literally "trying on" different implants. The doctor will show you a variety of implant "shells" — plastic sacs filled to different capacities with saline solution. You slip these into your bra to see their effect, trying on different sizes and discussing the options with the doctor. The doctor may also measure your breast to help determine which size would be the most effective and most complimentary to your figure.

This last idea — choosing an implant that's complimentary to your figure — is a very important one. Many women are so anxious to have larger breasts that they don't care about proportion. For many, choosing a breast size that matches up proportionately to the body isn't even a consideration. "The bigger the better" is a common attitude. If the size is too extreme, the skin may stretch so much that it can become almost paper-thin, which looks strange and unhealthy. I've seen cases in which women have asked for 800 cc of saline (about the size of two D cups sitting on top of one another), and the result is a thin-skinned breast with the implant right underneath the skin.

Shape is important too. The new, modern implants come in round, contour, and teardrop shapes. On a 22-year-old girl we might use a round one, which is closer to the shape of a young breast. On a woman of 40, roundness may not look quite natural, so we'd use the contour shape, which produces a full breast that doesn't look unnaturally round. A woman with some sagging might do better with a teardrop shape, which again, matches her natural shape. These choices are made with the patient's help, and we always recommend choosing an implant that is close to the most natural form.

Patients are encouraged to bring in a photograph of a topless model showing what they consider to be ideal breasts. Of course doctors can't promise an exact match, but we can often get very close in terms of size and shape.

Incisions

Several types of incisions can be made, and the doctor will help the patient with her choice. One type is made in the fold under the breast. Another can be made in the armpit, and a third kind runs along the top edge of the areola (the dark area around the nipple). Additionally, some doctors are placing breast implants through a tube inserted in the navel. The deflated implant is rolled up like a taco and moved up the tube into the breast, then inflated with the saline.

The armpit incision and the areola incision can leave a scar that may show, while the incision underneath the breast is generally better hidden. The navel incision is usually not apparent at all. "Keloid" or thick scars are a small risk in everyone, and a higher risk in patients with darker skin color. If this begins to occur after your surgery, get in to see your doctor as soon as possible. He should be able to improve your problem with injections of cortisone or silicone patches.

Implant Site

Implants can be inserted either behind the muscle or in front of it, between the muscle and the breast tissue. If the implant is placed in front of the muscle, there's less disturbance during surgery because only the soft tissue is being cut and manipulated to make room for the implant. Implants in front of the muscle may also look more dramatic, because they're closer to the surface and produce better cleavage and more projection. If a patient has enough breast tissue, which is a combination of fat and glandular tissue, then this may be the ideal position for the implant.

If a patient has very little breast tissue, it's preferable to put the implant behind the muscle. In this case, recovery is somewhat more difficult because the muscle layers have to be cut and separated. The good news is that if it's behind the muscle, the "rippling" effect that sometimes occurs with saline implants will be less visible. It also may look a little more natural when it's behind the muscle, because of the existing tissue on top of it. Finally, one of the possible complications of breast augmentation is that the breast can sometimes harden over time, as scar tissue forms around the implant. If the implant is placed behind the muscle, this hardening is less likely to occur.

How It's Done

When you arrive at the office, you'll be given a sedative, most likely Valium®, to help you relax. Once you're in the surgery room, you may also be given an intravenous drip of stronger medications. Most breast surgery today is still done under general anesthesia, but this isn't always necessary for doctors expert in tumescent anesthesia. If tumescent anesthetic is being used, it is injected at this point. This has the dual purpose of numbing the area and inhibiting bleeding (see chapter 15 on tumescent anesthesia). When tumescent is *not* used, there is more bleeding during surgery and more swelling and bruising during recovery. With general anesthetic and without tumescent, "cauterization" or electrical burning is often necessary to control bleeding.

If general anesthetic isn't used, you'll be sedated but not asleep. You'll be aware of what's going on around you, but you should feel little or no discomfort. The doctor will make an incision, usually about one-inch long (the navel incisions are smaller). Through this incision, the doctor will have access to the inside of the breast. With his fingers and with instruments, he will create a "pocket" either behind the muscle or behind the breast tissue. This is the most difficult part of the surgery, because the muscle and tissue are being pushed and stretched to make room for the implant, and this is why bruising occurs during the post-operative period.

Once the doctor makes the pocket and cleanses the opening, he inserts the implant shell. These shells, which are like thin plastic bubbles, come packaged and filled with air. The doctor first deflates the shell, and then inserts it flat into the pocket. Once it's in position, he fills it with saline solution, using a syringe connected to a tube leading into the shell. The breast puffs up like a balloon as the implant fills with saline.

When both breasts are filled, the doctor can make minor adjustments if needed. The table is cranked up so that the patient is in an upright position, allowing the doctor to look at her straight on to make sure the breasts look even. The incisions are left open so he can go back in and adjust the implants if necessary. When the doctor is satisfied with the appearance, the incision is closed in three layers. A first layer of absorbable stitches is made in the breast tissue. A second layer of absorbable stitches is put into the deeper layer of skin, and the third layer, of non-absorbable stitches, closes the outside skin. These outer stitches will be removed in about one week.

It all takes about 90 minutes. If you aren't completely asleep, you may be able to see your new breasts in a mirror when the doctor sits you up to take a look.

Mastopexy

In cases where the breast has become very droopy from childbirth, age, or genetic predisposition, women can opt to have a surgery called mastopexy. It's designed to lift the nipple up higher, by removing excess skin and literally raising up the entire breast.

Mastopexy involves several different incision options, some of which may leave quite a bit of scarring. The traditional incision is made in three parts: a circular cut that goes around the areola, a second incision running vertically from the areola to the fold underneath the breast, and a third incision across the fold. The cut looks like a keyhole, and it completely opens up the breast. In some cases, a "crescent mastopexy" can be done, in which the only incision is a small crescent at the top of the areola.

A more modern option, if appropriate for the patient, is to use only the circular cut around the areola. This separates the areola from the skin, enabling the doctor to cut away excess skin and tighten up the breast by pulling the skin together like a purse string, with a permanent suture. This lifts everything up and moves the nipple and areola to a higher position. Although the scar from this incision is not as obvious as the keyhole incision, it still may show. Fortunately, there is a process known as "tattooing," in which color that matches your skin color is literally tattooed into the scar. Another option is to return to the doctor's office a few months after surgery to have the scar treated by laser peeling (please see chapter 5 for a description of the laser peeling procedure).

Since most mastopexy patients don't have very much breast tissue, we'll often insert an implant at the same time to make the breast look fuller.

Breast Reduction

Many women seeking breast reduction may have physical or emotional problems because their breasts are too large for their bodies. Physically, the extra weight of the oversized breasts puts a strain on the back and can result in stooped posture, back pain, and more serious spinal problems. Emotionally, many women feel singled out socially because other people notice their breasts rather than their other qualities. I've heard many women say, "I'm having this surgery because I'm tired of people talking to my chest instead of to my face."

The surgery can also be done while you're awake, with sedation and tumescent anesthesia. However, most are done with general anesthetic. The incision options are the same as for mastopexy, but the keyhole incision is the one most commonly used. Reduction is accomplished by simply cutting away breast tissue and fat. If tumescent anesthetic is used, there is very little bleeding, and the whole procedure takes about two to three hours.

Because breasts have a good percentage of fat, it is also possible to do a reduction with liposuction. If a woman is a candidate for this — depending on several factors, including the elasticity of the skin and the size of the breast — she can lose a full cup size with lipo-suction alone. If you are considering breast reduction, be sure to ask your doctor about liposuction as an option. The extent of the doctor's liposuction expe-rience and whether you are a good candidate for the procedure are the key factors in a successful outcome.

Recovery

Recovery from breast augmentation is easier than recovery from mastopexy or breast reduction because the incision is so much smaller. You'll go home from the doctor's office wearing a special bra designed to hold the skin and muscles still, which has an effect similar to that of an ace bandage. This bra should be worn for at least six to eight weeks.

Tumescent anesthetic takes up to 24 hours to wear off and will minimize the pain during this period. Implants below the muscle are more painful and prescription pain killers are often needed for several days. Generally, implants above the muscle are much less uncomfortable. You may also be given an antibiotic to help decrease the possibility of infection.

You'll need to take it easy for a few days, and bed rest may be required after mastopexy or reduction. Strenuous exercise is out of the question for four to six weeks after augmentation, and six to eight weeks after mastopexy or reduction. You can take a shower and even go to work within a few days after augmentation if you're comfortable. But it's important that you don't lift your arms above shoulder level for the first couple of weeks after implants have been put in. They need time to settle into place, and the tissue needs a chance to start healing. Too much movement can move the implants or cause the incisions to open.

When you return home after augmentation, your breasts will be swollen and will feel tight and hard from the skin stretching. This effect is greater if tumescent is used. The swelling will decrease day by day, so the size of your breasts on the first day will be different than their final size. The feeling of tightness will also change as the skin stretches and loosens up. The entire shrinking and loosening process can take anywhere from two to six months or longer.

Results

Results are usually excellent. My patients often tell me that they have the breasts they've always wanted. Dissatisfaction is pretty rare, and is usually related to the size of the implants. It's hard to predict with complete certainty how a woman will feel with a new breast size, but dissatisfaction with breasts that are too large or too small can be easily fixed. With mastopexy and reduction, scarring can be a problem, but the patients are still generally happy, given proper counseling before the procedure.

Over the long term, there are no real rules to remember other than to wear a bra for support, even though with implants, it may not appear to be necessary. If you've had very large implants, the skin can stretch quite a bit from carrying all that extra weight and, if you haven't worn a bra for support, you'll have sagging. Gravity and age play their parts, and as you get older, some sagging will occur, as with the rest of the body.

The new saline implants have a tendency to "ripple," simply because they're filled with liquid, and when a woman bends or moves in certain ways, this rippling can be seen if the implants are placed behind the breast tissue. It's not usually noticeable, and most women don't mind it a bit. If the implant is placed behind the muscle, the rippling is less visible.

Numbness of the breasts occurs in less than five percent of patients. This happens because in the process of cutting away tissue, small nerves may be cut. However, these nerves heal themselves over time, and the numbness usually goes away. In very rare cases, even with the most competent and careful surgery, a major nerve may be involved, in which case numbness can last indefinitely. A decrease in nipple sensation occurs in about seven percent of patients when this area is used for the incision. Other rare complications include poor healing of the edges of an incision and the possibility of internal bleeding. But these can happen occasionally with *any* kind of invasive surgery, and they are extremely rare.

Occasionally, the breast may gradually harden after surgery as scar tissue forms. In some cases even 10 or

20 years later, scar tissue has to be removed. In the old days of silicone implants, hardening occurred in 15 percent of patients. With the new saline implants, the occurrence may be only two or three percent.

In some cases, there can be problems with shape or symmetry. This can often be corrected by changing the implants or adding or subtracting fluid from them. Keep in mind that absolute symmetry can never occur, because breasts (and faces and bodies) are naturally not perfectly even. Overall, 95 percent of our patients are delighted with their breast surgery results.

ɬ Patient Stories ℘

Leslie, age 21

I needed an implant because my left breast was about half the size of my right one, and it had been that way since puberty. It just didn't develop at the same rate as the right one, and it's been a terrible problem for me. I always had to wear an extra pad in my bra, and sew pads into bathing suits.

I spoke with many people before deciding on surgery, and that really helped to build up my confidence. I had the implant done about five weeks ago, and now the bruising's gone and the breast has shrunk down a bit, as they said it would. I think I look great. My breast doesn't have that fake look, that round line on top like so many that I've seen on movie stars and models. It looks real. When I wear a bathing suit, nobody can tell.

Karen, age 38

I'm a body builder, and when my breast muscles began to tighten up, I ended up basically flat-chested. Bench pressing causes the breast to turn into muscle, and it doesn't look feminine.

I had the surgery about five months ago. The recovery was difficult for me, because unlike most patients, my muscle tissue is really tough and tight, so cutting it and moving it around caused a lot of discomfort. But it was more than worth it.

Also, because I'm African American, they told me that scarring might be a problem (I had the incision around the nipple). But everything came out perfect. I couldn't be happier.

Terri, age 20

I didn't feel confident about myself, and I thought about having my breasts enlarged for a long time. But because I'm so young I figured I probably wouldn't do it until later. But then I just decided to go through with it, and even though there was bruising and some pain afterwards, I'm totally happy that I did it, and I'd recommend it to anyone. I went from an A to a C cup. The best part was going shopping for new bras.

Hair Transplantation

    ☞ *Hair transplantation takes hair from the back of the head where "permanent" hair grows, and transplants it to the balding front. This "donor hair" will stay and grow, just like it would have in the back.*

    ☞ *The methods for doing this have improved vastly in recent years, with much better results, less patient discomfort and less recovery time.*

    ☞ *There are currently no good alternatives for hair transplantation except hairpieces, which have many disadvantages.*

    ☞ *The modern procedure is done under local anesthetic and takes four to eight hours.*

    ☞ *After the first 10 days, not much is seen in the transplanted area. Usually new hair growth takes four months.*

Hair transplantation has been practiced for decades, and the results have been mixed. But recent innovations are downright *revolutionary.*

Results have improved more in the last five years than in the prior 20. The old pluggy, toothbrushy look is gone. When skillfully done, today's transplants are virtually indistinguishable from a normal hair pattern. The doctors who have changed with the times are seeing superb results, and the ones who still use the old methods are getting compromised or mediocre results.

How It's Done

Hair transplantation involves removing some of the hair-bearing scalp from the back of the head and planting it in the front of the head in tiny seedlings or "grafts." The hair continues to grow in the front just as it was doing in the back (the "permanent hair" from the back of the head generally grows life-long). The area from which the hair is removed at the back of the head is called the "donor site." This is closed with stitches or staples, generally heals quickly, and is concealed with the remaining hair. The staples are usually removed in 10 to 14 days.

In the last few years doctors have used smaller and smaller graft sizes. In the past, large "plugs" — groups of up to 25 hair roots — were transplanted together, but now the tiny grafts contain just one to six hairs. We've learned that fewer hairs per graft produce a more natural result, and the problem of handling large numbers of grafts has also been solved. The techniques for "harvesting" hair from the back of the head have improved too. These new techniques result in less damage to the remaining hair, less healing time, less discomfort, and a better look.

Alternatives to transplantation aren't great. Hairpieces are a hassle. They're expensive (generally more than transplants over the long term), they don't look natural, and they can come off or move out of place unexpectedly, causing terrible embarrassment. And some physicians think that hairpieces actually kill more hair. The only other alternative, Rogaine®, is a nonprescription hair growth medicine applied to the scalp. It's relatively expensive and works for only about 25 percent of users. And, if you stop using it, any new hair will fall out. So transplantation is rapidly gaining popularity. Most "new hair" seen on the heads of American men these days involves the minor surgery of hair transplantation.

Who are our Patients?

In my experience working with hair transplant patients, it's clear that some men are critically affected by their hair loss. Hair is vital to an individual's self esteem, and this message has been expressed to us in literature and advertising for centuries.

Most hair transplant patients are men between the ages of 30 and 50, but in some cases, men as young as 25 will come in for consultations if their hair loss has already begun. Hair transplants in younger men are problematic, however, because the hair loss pattern hasn't completely declared itself. Physicians need to allow for the natural elevation of the hairline that will continue to occur in the years to come. If we transplant hair too low in the front, it will create a look that's too young — an odd looking hairline for a mature man.

You may be surprised to learn that women also suffer from hair loss. Over 200,000 people had hair transplants in 1994 (more than four times the 1990 rate), and among them, about 13,000 were women.

On the Day of Your Procedure

When you arrive at the office or surgical center, your doctor will mark the outline of your new hairline. As you get older, and your hairline continues to recede, you'll want the new one to be appropriate *for your age*. If it's placed too low, similar to where it was when you were 20 years old, it will look quite strange and inappropriate when you are 50 or 60.

After this, you'll be given a relaxation medicine, and the process will begin. Many of our patients sleep for 20 to 40 minutes and "miss" most of the procedure. They don't feel a thing.

The doctor will closely examine the back of the head, or the "donor" area, and will count hair density with a magnifying instrument. Based on the number of the grafts to be planted, he will decide how big an area needs work.

Next, the area is numbed, and the donor hair is removed. You may feel a little pressure during this process, but little or no pain. This donor site on the back of the head heals with a linear scar that is usually only visible to your hairdresser.

Once this process is complete, the patient sleeps or watches television while the technicians divide the donor hair into tiny segments, sometimes as small as a quarter of a grain of rice. The smallest segments contain only one or two hairs. These are the grafts, and they're being prepared to "plant" into tiny openings on the head. Each one becomes part of the new scalp and will grow in naturally. They're cut into just the right size so that a "toothbrush" look does not occur when the hair starts to grow. There are from one to four hairs in each graft, in most cases.

While the technicians are working, the doctor numbs the scalp and makes tiny openings where the grafts are to be inserted. It's a lot like transplanting seedlings in a garden. The openings are made at the proper angle so that the hair grows correctly. In the front of the head the hair grows forward and somewhat to the sides, and in the back of the head it grows backward. Sometimes the doctor can even reproduce the irregular pattern or "whorl" that occurs in the crown. There is generally no discomfort during the procedure (the local anesthetic works like a charm). You can be awake and chatting with the doctor and technicians, or possibly a little sleepy from the relaxation medicine.

A typical hair transplant session involves 1,200 to 1,500 grafts and sometimes more. It's a long, slow process, inserting the grafts one at a time with small forceps. A thousand is a good number for both our technicians and patients — no one gets too tired, and patients are impressed with the quantity of hair they ultimately get. Some doctors do more grafts per session, but there is controversy about graft survival with the higher numbers. The grafts fit snugly into the openings, and the skin simply seals together. Because these hairs were taken from the back of the head where the "permanent" hair grows, the newly transplanted hair will remain intact as long as the hair at the donor site does. Generally, this is life-long.

When you schedule your hair transplant, plan on spending anywhere from three to ten hours in the doctor's office or surgical center. A proper modern hair transplant is a labor-intensive process, and implanting tiny grafts into over a thousand points on the scalp takes time.

It isn't usually necessary to have anyone drive you home after the procedure. You should recover in a couple of hours and be able to drive yourself home safely. With the new-style tiny grafts, you can resume relatively normal activities the next day with no problems. It might be better to avoid heavy exercise for several days. There's no need to take time off from work or from your routine social activities. With the older style hair plugs, you had to be careful to avoid a lot of activity for fear of losing the grafts, which were four millimeters in diameter thick. Now, you'll just have some redness of your scalp, and possibly some scabbing, which will last for 10 days or less.

What About Scalp Surgery for Hair Loss?

"Scalp reductions" or "lifts" consist of cutting out bald skin from the top of the head and stretching the hairy "sidewall" up over the crown. Some doctors are even doing complex surgery to take strips of hair from the sides of the head, swinging them into the front, and stitching them in place. While these might sound like good ideas, they should be weighed carefully in view of the new techniques. To completely understand the change in medical thinking, you need education as a hair transplant doctor. But as an overview:

- The front of any natural hairline is very complex and wispy, with a critical forward-leaning hair direction. It can't be imitated by a dense "flap."

- The new hair transplantation is very labor-intensive and needs a team of expert technicians to painstakingly reconstruct the frontal hairline. Some of the old-style doctors haven't been able to put together the collective expertise to do the new transplants.

- Severe and visible scarring is common with incisional scalp surgery.

- We now know what happens to the scalp over the long term, after more natural hair loss occurs. *It very often looks terrible 10 years later! I must* put it in these terms, for the doctors who persist with this surgery are ignoring the long term for a short term result, and are probably doing it merely for financial gain. The scars and the subsequent hair loss patterns are frequently awful-looking.

These aren't just my opinions. Dr. Mario Marzola, for example, is internationally famous among hair transplant doctors. He has specialized for decades in scalp surgery and has a surgical procedure named after him, the "Marzola Flap and "Marzola Lateral Lift". At a recent international conference, he showed photo after photo of his very bad results after five to ten years. With great courage and honesty he said, "The Marzola Flap and the Lateral Lift are dead. I believe they should not be performed again. I have stopped performing them." And as Dow Stough, M.D., former president of the International Society of Hair Restoration Surgery said recently, "A significant number of scalp reduction patients are dissatisfied, regardless of the surgeon. I believe that those surgeons who deny this fact spring from the ostrich-with-his-head-in-the-sand syndrome. They simply don't want to know the down side."

The unnatural effects of scalp surgery are often obvious even to a lay person. Men who wear hats to conceal their baldness will frequently wear hats after scalp lifting to conceal their post-surgical look.

Recovery

When you leave the office, you may have a headband and bandages around your head to protect the donor site. The majority of patients have little trouble sleeping the first night, and any discomfort can be relieved with prescription medications. Patients having second and third procedures sometimes have a little more postoperative discomfort.

Most patients find it convenient to return to the doctor the next day to have their dressings removed and their hair washed. Some are instructed to remove their own dressings if they live a long distance from the office. You won't need any kind of bandage after this point, and the grafts won't usually be very obvious, other than some redness or crusting. Any shampooing you do should be done gently. Scabbing can last up to 10 days. You should stay out of the sun, and if you live or work in an environment that's dusty or dirty, you should wear a cap.

The doctor will recheck you in 10 days to remove stitches from the donor area. After the first month you may see about a quarter inch of hair growth, but it's just as likely that the hair may go into a dormant period for about two to three months after surgery, and then start growing again. This is normal, and doesn't mean that the transplant didn't "take." At about four months, you will often see a quarter to a half inch of hair. The hair gradually thickens and strengthens over a period of about 12 months.

Results

It's important that you do not expect your hair to return to 100 percent of its original glory. But the improvements after a hair transplant can be very impressive, and it *will* grow. Realistic expectations are vital to your satisfaction. Yes, we *do* replace thousands of hairs, and you *will* have real, natural hair growing in an area that may once have had little or none. But keep in mind that hair transplantation is also somewhat of a visual trick, designed to make it look like you have more hair than you really have. So don't expect the same density that you have in the back of your head.

In many cases, a patient may wish to return for additional transplants several months after the first surgery (some doctors graft again in six weeks, but we believe that this may kill hair). When large quantities of hair need to be implanted, repeat sessions can be scheduled every four to six months. Some patients who are persistent with their process sometimes have five or even ten sessions, but this is unnecessary with the large number of grafts transplanted using modern methods. More commonly, men are very satisfied with 2,000 to 3,000 grafts for an area of baldness that extends over the whole top of the scalp. If you have some hair to begin with, you may need fewer grafts.

ও Patient Stories ৶

Bob, age 54

I was 52 when I had my hair transplant done. All my life I had a beautiful full crop of hair, and it was very important to me. When I started losing it in front, in typical male pattern baldness, a friend of mine at the gym told me about his doctor. I met with him, and I felt very comfortable — there was a real personal connection there.

I feel fantastic about the results. I ask my friends to tell me honestly how it looks, and they say that they can't even tell that I've had anything done. They're used to seeing bad transplants on other people, the kind that look like little squares of hair on people's heads. Mine doesn't look like that at all. It looks great.

Bart, age 35

I'm the youngest of four brothers, and all of us have lost our hair. One of my older brothers had a hair transplant years ago, and it was just a horror story. It looked terrible. You could see the plugs of hair sticking out all over his head. I decided to wait a few years before looking into doing my own, hoping that doctors would develop better ways of doing it.

When micro grafting finally came around, I was interested, but I couldn't afford it. I still shopped around though, but I found most of the doctors I talked to had real bad attitudes, and their offices were like assembly lines, very impersonal. I finally found someone I trusted and who I thought would do a good job.

I had two sessions, and I'm really happy with my results. The last procedure was about three months ago, and I can see that about 50 percent of the hairs are already growing.

Vein Therapy 12

  Large veins are best treated with surgery, and small veins with injection.

  The new large-vein removal techniques are easy, comfortable and safe compared to the old style "stripping."

  Complications for these procedures if performed in the modern manner are exceedingly rare.

  Patients frequently report relief of aching legs after either injection or surgery.

Vein surgery is one of the most common cosmetic procedures performed in the United States. Nearly half a million individuals had vein surgery every year in the mid 1990s. As technology advances and the surgery becomes simpler and more risk-free, the numbers continue to increase.

The vast majority of people with vein problems are women, particularly those who've been pregnant. Veins get worse with second pregnancies, though we're really not sure why. Heredity, weight gain, and hormones all seem to play a role.

Until the last few years, the only option for the treatment of unsightly and uncomfortable varicose veins was major surgery requiring general anesthesia, sometimes involving a hospital stay of several days. It was a big procedure, which involved making as many as ten incisions of one-half to one inch in length and vigorously removing the veins with large instruments.

It was a brutal process compared to modern methods, and the recovery period was longer and more difficult. Patients were often advised to have extended bed rest, as severe bruising occurred and infections were more frequent.

In the last few years, however, new therapies have improved on the major surgical procedure. "Sclerotherapy," or injection therapy, is a minor procedure that is easily done in a physician's office and has become commonplace. Vein removal using new "hooking techniques" with tumescent anesthetic (please read about tumescent anesthetic in chapter 15) is a relatively minor procedure usually done in an outpatient surgical center. In either case, the patient is generally up and on her feet a few hours after the procedure. Sclerotherapy is most effective for smaller veins (less than one eighth of an inch in diameter), while hooking is used for larger veins. Scarring is minimal compared to the old procedure.

People seek help for vein problems when visual clues, such as bulging veins, brown pigment and possibly even a firmer surface of the surrounding skin, indicate that the system isn't functioning properly. Veins carry the blood through the body and back to the heart. They have valves every inch or so, which keep the blood flowing in the proper direction. When these valves become defective, the blood is not conveyed back to the heart efficiently. Instead, the blood will "pool," and this generally occurs in the legs because they're lowest and subjected to a long column of pressure. This can cause cosmetic problems —varicose and spider veins are not pretty. But in some cases, circulatory problems can occur, which cause aching legs. In the worst cases, circulation can be seriously affected and the leg severely damaged or destroyed.

The beauty of vein treatments is that they can simply *eliminate* bad veins, which will then free the entire system to start running smoothly again. There are many, many extra veins, and the normal healthy ones simply take over when the bad ones are removed.

Preparation

Candidates for vein procedures are generally childbearing age and older. After pregnancy, especially a second pregnancy, veins may get worse. Vein treatments are relatively simple procedures, and there are not many situations in which a patient would be advised against it. Women who are taking birth control pills are one exception because, in rare cases, this can contribute to clotting problems. In cases where a patient already has a clotting disorder, it may not be advisable to treat the veins. Also, women should not be treated during pregnancy.

If you are being treated for large veins using vein hooking, you may need to take one to two days off from work. Plan to wear compression socks for about a week, usually with a wrap over this for the first 12 to 24 hours. You may walk normally after your procedure, but long backpacking trips are out for at least a week. It's a good idea to plan on having someone drive you home from the surgical center if you've had relaxation medicines. In many cases, however, no medication besides the local anesthetics is needed. Make sure you have loose comfortable clothes that will fit over any bandages.

If you're having sclerotherapy, you can return to work the same day. There are no drugs or anesthetic given, and you'll have no problem driving yourself home. You'll probably be wearing some kind of support stocking.

How It's Done

Vein Hooking

Removing large varicose veins, back in the days when it was done in a hospital under general anesthesia, used to involve making incisions about one inch long, threading a long wire through the incision and through the vein from the groin to the knee, hooking the vein onto the wire, and pulling the whole thing out. This caused a lot of bleeding and bruising, and physicians often advised one or two weeks of bed rest, which had the potential to cause circulatory problems because the patient was immobile for so long. Despite the new alternatives, this method is still commonly used.

The new methods are an entirely different story. For anesthesia, we use the same tumescent anesthetic that we use for liposuction, which numbs the area and decreases bleeding. The technique for hooking the vein is similar, but the instrument is smaller, and instead of pulling the entire vein out, we remove it in small segments of up to six inches long. Since the vein was already dysfunctional, the circulation system simply compensates for its removal by channeling the blood through the thousands of other working veins.

The leg has two major veins, either of which can be varicose and need removal. One begins at the groin and is seen on the entire inside of the leg. Another is located at the back of the knee, appearing on the upper calf. Several other leg vein systems may be dysfunctional and need to be removed as well. Tiny incisions are made wherever the veins bulge, and they are hooked out with our new tiny specialized tools. If the valves for the large groin vein are not working properly, they will frequently be tied at the groin, cutting off their connection to the rest of the system. This is called "flush ligation." The incision is made in the groin crease, where the scar is less visible.

The entire procedure usually takes between one and three hours, and the patient feels little or no discomfort.

Sclerotherapy

Sclerotherapy can be used on the larger veins I've described above, but the results may be only temporary, with a good chance of recurrence within two years. Sclerotherapy is best used for small spider veins.

When you arrive at the office for sclerotherapy, you'll be put into an examining room and asked to put on a gown. There is no anesthetic necessary. You will have photographs taken and be given a consent form that describes the unlikely but possible complications.

The doctor will then inject your spider veins with a tiny needle, almost the smallest ever used in clinical practice, so small and sharp that most people barely feel it. Using magnifying glasses and a good light, the doctor injects solution into the "feeder system" of veins that runs underneath the obvious spider veins. The spiders can also be injected directly, but I feel that the feeder method gives the best results. Depending on the number of areas injected, the procedure can take anywhere from 10 to 30 minutes. There is no bleeding or pain, and you'll walk out of the doctor's office with nothing more than an ace bandage or a compression stocking. Some doctors use no compression, but best results are probably obtained with support socks worn right after the procedure.

Several injection sessions are generally needed to get the best result, depending on your particular veins and the doctor's skill.

Recovery

After you leave the office, you'll likely be wearing a compression stocking, possibly covered with an ace bandage. There may be leakage of tumescent fluid if you've had a vein hooking procedure, and this will have a pink tinge or red color. This is not blood, but rather the fluid mixed with a tiny amount of blood.

After vein hooking, you can resume limited normal activity as soon as you leave the office. What you *don't* want to do is to completely immobilize yourself. It's important to keep active in order to keep the blood flowing. Normal activity, like walking, light bike riding, and housework is not only fine, but recommended. Don't overdo it — mountain climbing is out for a while. You'll be wearing a bandage or compression socks for a week, even in the shower (you can cover it with plastic to keep it dry). When you take the bandage off, the big veins are usually gone. You may have a few fragments left, which can be treated with sclerotherapy during your follow-up visits.

After sclerotherapy you can do whatever you want. You'll usually be given compression stockings to wear during your waking hours for several days. When you remove these, you may see hard and ropy-looking veins, but don't worry — they're generally on their way out. You may also see bruising, which most frequently lasts a few weeks. Skin discoloration can occasionally persist for months or even be permanent for a rare patient, but it almost always looks much better than the veins. But while all this is going on, you will see the veins disappearing, which should make you feel great. You probably want to look for that old mini skirt in the back of the closet.

Results and Complications

In simple terms, the results are better looking legs, but of course this depends on what you had to begin with. A 70 percent improvement is a good result, and the vast majority of our patients are very happy. However, we do tell our patients that injection therapy is like going to the dentist; they may have to come back every several years for a touch-up. The vein hooking procedures are usually more permanent.

A rare complication with injection, seen less than one percent of the time, is skin ulceration. I've seen just one in my whole experience. These heal with a flat, small scar. Blood clots that go to the lungs or cause serious problems with circulation occur rarely with vein hooking using tumescent anesthetic, and are almost unheard of with injection. Many vein doctors work full time for years and never see a complication like a serious blood clot.

⪦ Patient Stories ⪧

Marsha, age 61

I decided to have the procedure because my legs were tired all the time. I had a hard time standing, and I wore support stockings. Some

---

of my veins were so bad that it looked like they were going to pop out of my legs.

My doctor said I was a good candidate for injections and the removal of the large veins. So I did it, and now I'm so happy because my legs are no longer tired. The recovery was easy, not bad at all. I didn't have to stay off my feet or anything. I just wore support stockings for about a week, and that was it. My legs look 100 percent better.

Danielle, age 34

I had tiny little spider veins, and a few bigger ones here and there. I'd had liposuction about a year earlier, and my thighs were shaped beautifully. But the veins were still there, and it didn't make sense to have gone to all that trouble to get rid of the fat and not get rid of the veins too. So about a year after the lipo, I had sclerotherapy — where they inject the little veins with saline solution and they simply dissolve. It really worked. The veins pretty much disappeared.

Marguerite, age 60

I had very large varicose veins, and as I got older, my legs began to ache terribly. I wasn't so concerned about the way they looked, though they looked awful, but I'd heard that having them treated might make my legs feel better. Looking better was an added plus. It's been two years, I can walk more comfortably, and I'm not ashamed of how my thighs look when I wear shorts.

A Word about Cellulite

13

Some of this material was contributed by Dr. Riad Roomi, a plastic surgeon practicing in London, England

꿍 *Cellulite is treatable! Massage, ultrasound, and a new French roller machine all may produce benefits.*

Cellulite, a word popularized in the 1970s and 80s, describes the phenomenon of "dimpled fat," which is the bane of female thighs. As best doctors can tell, cellulite occurs because the skin is tethered down by strings of tissue pulling it inward, toward the interior of the body. These strings pull sections of fat in along with them. It's not unlike the way a mattress has dimples due to the strings holding the "tucks" down.

Cellulite seems to begin in puberty in women due to hormonal changes. Some degree of cellulite is found on almost every woman over 18 years of age. Age, genetics, family history and racial factors all play a role. Dark-skinned women tend to be less "cellulitic" than light-skinned women, though we're not exactly sure why this is.

The cellulite fat can be removed by liposuction, and the strings of tissue can be cut by scraping under the surface of the skin to disconnect them from their hold on the fat. This works best in younger patients, and older patients occasionally get skin changes after liposuction that may be similar to cellulite. It varies with the individual.

Massage *can* be effective if performed very, very vigorously — even painfully hard. This can leave bruising over the first several sessions until the patient's body becomes used to it. After 10 to 20 sessions, people usually begin to show results. But it isn't for everyone. It's time consuming, painful, and the results depend a lot on the type of fat you have. Very soft fat — usually found in older patients and in people with lighter skins — seems to respond better, but it's hard to find a masseuse who can rub hard enough to separate the fat from the "strings." In terms of new medical developments, there are currently some European specialists who've gotten positive publicity for their work with ultrasonic cellulite treatments combined with massage and brushing of the skin. The treatments can require as many as 20 to 40 sessions, but they appear to be quite effective. There's also an expensive new French instrument that looks like a big vacuum cleaner for your thighs. It pulls on the cellulite areas and supposedly smoothes everything out. My understanding is that this $25,000 vacuum cleaner works about as well as massage, but requires a similar amount of patience to endure 20 to 40 treatments. We are currently using a simple vacuum method that sucks a 3½-inch circle of skin into a cup. This seems to work as well as anything else. A good diet, lots of fluids, and compression girdles are helpful, too.

Just how long these manipulation-based methods last is open to debate; the masseuses say they must maintain their results by on-going weekly massage. I suspect that some of the improvement is due to swelling — the flat area rises to meet the raised area. My personal feeling is that liposuction produces a quicker, better, longer lasting result.

❧ Patient Stories ☙

Dorothy, age 57

Since early adulthood I've had dimpled thighs, and I'd been very self-conscious about it most of my life. With some weight gain after I went through menopause, I noticed a change for the worse. I finally decided to do something about it, and went to the doctor for liposuction. It was greatly improved (I was down two dress sizes) but there was still a lot of irregularity. The doctor suggested that I try massage and ultrasound.

The masseuse was rough and the process was a little painful, especially the first three sessions. I got some bruises until I toughened up. My treatment lasted twice a week for 32 sessions total — but the results were worth it. My knees and thighs can be shown off. I don't look like I'm 22, but I'm not ashamed any more, and I can wear skirts with hose. The results have lasted six months now without any more treatments.

The Lowdown on Lasers 14

> ⚡ *Several new expensive lasers are now being used for many different skin problems.*

> ⚡ *Excess hair, tattoos, and red spots can be effectively treated.*

> ⚡ *Other problems may often be treated less expensively with traditional technology.*

The amount of hype and advertising about laser surgery is overwhelming. What's the real truth and the real role of lasers in cosmetic surgery?

What is a laser?

The term "laser" is actually an acronym for Light Amplification by Stimulated Emission of Radiation. In simple terms, a laser tool emits a beam of light which, when focused on the skin, will "vaporize" — or disintegrate — its target. In many ways, the concept seems straight out of a science fiction movie. The beam of light is actually sensitive to different colors of the spectrum, which is why lasers can remove colored areas on the skin, such as brown spots and tattoos. There are many different types of lasers "tuned" to different color frequencies, and other types designed specifically for resurfacing skin by vaporization of everything down to a certain depth.

The most important advance in the field of laser surgery is skin resurfacing (please see chapter 5 on facial laser peeling for a complete description of this procedure). Carbon Dioxide and Erbium lasers have supplanted the old style chemical (acid) peeling and dermabrasion for the removal of wrinkles and facial scars. Although there are several brand names for the CO_2 lasers, at this writing the Coherent Ultra Pulse has the most advanced technology. Coherent has a research budget alone that's larger than the total revenues of many of its competitors.

A recent development is the "scanning" laser, which scans a focused beam across a larger area of skin than the older lasers were able to cover. Scanners can treat an area of possibly $1/2$ to $3/4$ of an inch in diameter in less than a second. Without these scanners, only small areas ($1/8$ to $1/10$ of an inch) could be zapped at a time. It used to take hours to treat the whole face this way, and uneven results were not uncommon. Scanners made resurfacing much faster and more accurate.

The newest player in the facial resurfacing arena is the Erbium laser. Similar to the Carbon Dioxide laser, this laser reacts with the water moisture in the skin to create a vaporization effect, but that is where the similarities end. The Erbium laser, or "cold laser" at it is sometimes called, treats the skin in much smaller increments, allowing for finer control of the resurfacing. Moreover, this laser creates much less heat damage than the CO_2 laser. This usually allows for faster post-op healing time and faster disappearance of the "red face" of healing often seen with resurfacing. The trade-off may be less wrinkle and scar removal than with the CO_2 lasers. Lastly, the Erbium allows the surgeon to perform this procedure on darker skin types, like those with olive to light brown skin tones.

What Lasers Can Do

Most people think of lasers in terms of facial skin resurfacing, but there are many other surprising medical and cosmetic uses. Here's an overview:

Tattoo Removal

Lasers which are sensitive to the different colors are used to remove tattoos. The lasers used are the Q-Switched Yag, the Q-Switched Ruby, and the Q-Switched Alexandrite. All three lasers can remove the dark blue/black inks, but only the Ruby and the Alexandrite can fade the green colors. The Yag can fade red inks, but the Ruby cannot. So if you have a multicolored tattoo to remove, make sure your doctor has access to at least two of these lasers.

Laser tattoo removal works by delivering extremely high energy and shattering the tattoo ink particle without destroying the surrounding skin. The reason a tattoo remains on the skin is because the pigment granules are so large that the body can't disperse them. The laser uses the wave length of the pigment and breaks the particles apart to help the body absorb it. Tattoo removal usually takes between four to ten sessions, with four to six weeks between sessions. Sometimes complete tattoo removal isn't possible. These procedures have a very high rate of patient satisfaction, but side effects sometimes include a change in skin texture or pigment.

Red Marks on the Face or Body

The lasers that treat "vascular" or abnormal blood vessels and red "birthmarks" on the skin surface represent a genuine advance. The flash lamp pulsed dye laser works well on Port Wine Stain birthmarks (the Gorbachov birthmark), cherry angiomas, and small hemangiomas or red spots. Sometimes many sessions are required, but usually very little scarring results after the work is done.

Pigment Irregularities

Using a laser that responds to color, age spots and other irregularities on hands or face can often be removed in a few sessions without scarring. The Q-Switched Yag and Q-Switched Alexandrite lasers remove freckles, moles, and age or sun spots. They can also fade and improve the appearance of brown birthmarks such as Becker's Nevus and Nevus of Ota. The Q-Switched Ruby, one of the most powerful lasers in medicine, also comes in handy for stubborn spots and birthmarks. While there may be bruising for five to seven days afterward, generally the spots disappear completely.

Tattooed Eyeliner Removal

This is done the same way as removal of other tattoos, but steel eye covers are placed over the eyes for protection. These lasers can also work on cosmetic eyebrow tattoos and tattooed lip liner. While cosmetologists have ways to correct or remove cosmetic tattoos, some of their methods may interfere with laser tattoo removal which might be needed in the future. We recommend you check with a laser center first before getting any cosmetic tattoo corrected or removed.

Sealing Broken Blood Vessels in the Face

There are two or three types of lasers used for this procedure. A pulse laser is often used, which emits quick pulses of light that are absorbed by certain chemicals (oxyhemoglobin) in the blood. Color sensitive lasers can also be used, or a combination of both. For broken blood vessels, lasers with lower energy are recommended because they are less aggressive with the already-damaged vessels.

Another good choice for treating broken capillaries on the face is the KTP 532nm laser. The KTP can seal broken capillaries on one's nose, resulting in up to 85 percent improvement which is visible instantly. You could even go to work the same day, since the treated area does not bruise.

Stretch Marks and Scars

Pulse lasers are used to improve stretch marks and scars, including acne scars. They may actually stimulate the cells to make collagen, which helps flat areas rise to meet the raised areas. A 40 to 70 percent improvement in stretch marks is possible in some cases. Darkening of the skin can outweigh the benefits in darker skinned patients.

For scars, the best results have been obtained when laser treatment begins as soon as possible after a scar has formed. Cortesone injection is often used when treating a scar at this early stage. Dermatologists are usually the most skilled at using just the right amount of cortesone. Too much can cause actual depression of the scar.

Leg Veins

Specialized lasers for veins seal off the smaller vessels, but don't work for large varicose veins or on darker skin. One of the latest FDA-approved lasers for leg veins is the long-pulse Alexandrite. It can help remove veins between .6 to 2.0 millimeter in diameter. Generally the best results occur when injection is also used.

Hair Removal

This is a genuine advance, and there are several promising competitors, all claiming permanent or near-permanent hair removal. With some lasers there is no pain and almost no chance of scarring or other complications. The ideal treatment hasn't been found yet, but a replacement for the painful and tedious process of electrolysis will be reality soon.

In August 1997, the FDA approved the Cynosure Photogenica LPIR, a long-pulse Alexandrite laser which underwent almost two years of careful studies before its release. Results using this laser have been exceptional. These new Alexandrite systems are very quick and less painful than the previous laser hair removal systems. On average, after three to four treatments one experiences long-term relief from annoying hair growth. Laser hair removal is becoming the most convenient and economical way to remove hair from large sections of the body as well as from the face, underarms, and bikini areas.

Lasers are unbelievably expensive to own and operate. They cost anywhere from $30,000 to $250,000 (vision correction lasers cost $500,000!), and some doctors own several, with up to a million dollars invested in their equipment. The technology changes so rapidly that in a few short years the equipment becomes outmoded and has to be replaced. Is this expense really necessary to treat skin problems?

No, not always. We already have inexpensive ways to treat some of these problems. In some cases, such as skin resurfacing, hair removal, red "birthmark" treatment, and tattoo removal, the lasers represent a genuine advance. We just couldn't get the same quality of results and low complication rates with the conventional techniques. But for some conditions, the advantages of the laser are subtle.

What is Tumescent Anesthetic?

☙ *Tumescent anesthetic makes surgery safer, usually more accurate, and results in easier recoveries. It can be used for most cosmetic surgery.*

I believe that tumescent anesthetic is one of the main miracles of cosmetic surgery in the 1990s. Without it, we would not be able to perform many of the procedures described in this book as comfortable in-office surgeries. Without it, many procedures would necessitate additional expense for an anesthesiologist and possible side effects of general anesthesia, such as nausea and vomiting. Without tumescent, there would be more bleeding during surgery, more post-operative discomfort, and more bruising during recovery.

Tumescent anesthesia is a liquid solution which is injected *into the fat tissue* located directly under the skin. It's taken into the rest of the body slowly, and provides a localized effect. It's *not* injected into the bloodstream as many other types of anesthesia are.

Tumescent anesthesia's primary active ingredient is lidocaine, a standard anesthetic which numbs the area into which it's injected. It's similar to the novocaine that was once used in dentist's offices (they use lidocaine now). The numbing sensation you feel in your mouth when you have a tooth filled is the same kind of numbing you feel with tumescent. The lidocaine is mixed with a salt water solution similar to your body fluids.

A second medicine called adrenaline is added to the lidocaine solution. This is a "vasoconstrictor," a chemical which causes blood vessels to constrict, or close down. When the vessels are closed, less blood flows through them, so there's less bleeding during the surgery. Adrenaline is also known by the name epinephrine.

The mix of lidocaine and adrenaline is varied by different doctors for different procedures. The concentration we use for liposuction has just a small amount of active ingredients per volume of salt water, just enough to numb the fat and minimize bleeding. For hair transplants, we use more adrenaline, because the scalp has a lot more blood vessels and needs more constriction to prevent bleeding. For facial surgery, we again use a slightly different concentration of lidocaine and adrenaline.

We often use tumescent in combination with other medicines. For example, in many cases, when preparing patients for surgery, we'll give them a sedative such as Valium® to help them relax. This is very important because most patients are nervous. Many times we'll also give an intravenous pain reliever like Demerol® to relax them even further. This helps them to be less aware of what's going on around them, and enables them to drift off to sleep if they choose. One of the key advantages of keeping the patient relatively awake is that he or she can position for the doctor so the doctor can see just what is happening to the "sculpture" during the procedure. The patient can even stand up at the end of the case to check how good the result is. This isn't possible when general anesthetic is used.

When the tumescent fluid is injected into several sites of the area to be treated, it spreads throughout the fat tissue, numbing everything in its path and constricting the blood vessels. Because it's a liquid, it literally fills up the area under the skin, creating a bloated look. After the surgery, the remaining fluid which was not suctioned out drains through whatever openings were made in the skin. This drainage is mixed with a small amount of blood, which tinges the fluid with a pink or light red color. Many patients are concerned when they see this drainage, because they think they're bleeding. This is not the case. It's just the tumescent fluid draining out, with a few drops of blood mixed in. Without tumescent, there would be *real* bleeding.

Because the adrenaline inhibits bleeding, the tumescent technique also produces less bruising (a bruise is just blood collected under the skin). In the past, before tumescent, bruising could last a month after liposuction. Many cosmetic surgeons still don't use tumescent anesthesia, and their patients experience more bruising, longer recovery times, and even occasional blood transfusions.

Tumescent is taking a while to catch on in the medical community, as do most new techniques, but it's an amazing tool. When used properly, it is one of the safest ways to operate. The next chapter describes these safety issues.

What's the Worst That Can Happen? 16

- ℞ Read this critical chapter *before* you have surgery.
- ℞ *Any* surgery of *any* kind involves the risk of problems, even with the best of care.
- ℞ Don't expect your interaction with the doctor to end on the day of the surgery. You need proper follow up to get the best results.

Complications — a doctor's life would be so much easier without them, and they happen with statistical regularity to *anyone* who has surgery. Infections, bruising, fluid collections, imperfect results, slow healing, and other irritating complications are just *unavoidable* in a few patients.

Doing surgery isn't like changing the oil in a car. People all heal differently and surgery can be done in many different ways. Slight variations in technique can produce big problems (or more beautiful results) for different people. A doctor who claims that he never has problems with his patients is either inexperienced or a liar.

Cosmetic surgery is often a trade-off between good results and potential for problems. *Read this last sentence again. It is a key concept.* In other words, your chance for the best possible result may be related to how much surgery you have, and with more surgery, there is more chance of a problem. For example, with a face peel, the chance of *scarring* and the removal of wrinkles is increased with deeper peeling. The doctor has to judge just where to stop. This is easier with the laser than with the old acid peels or dermabrasion, but variables such as skin thickness and infection may change the result. **There's just no way to do any surgery in a perfectly exact way to get perfect results every time without any risk of problems.**

Liposuction gives us another example. With lipo, the chance of unattractive skin changes and even skin death increases with the amount of fat removed. But the doctor must take enough off to create a pleasing figure. *It's a trade-off between risk and benefit.*

What patients should understand when they sign on for cosmetic surgery is that they are committing to a *relationship* and a *process*. It's not like going to the restaurant and eating dinner. The transaction doesn't end on the day of the surgery. Out of 100 patients, perhaps 90 might be able to ignore the doctor's advice to be seen after surgery and they would heal just fine. For the other 10, follow-up might be important to insure the best result (these numbers aren't exact). For example, anti-inflammatory injections might be needed over a period of a couple of months. Some other patients might require extensive follow-up over a six to eight month period, or need a simple surgical procedure to correct the result.

One patient out of the hundred might be in for a long, bothersome hassle. She might have an infection, which would require going to the office for shots every day for a week. She might need a major revision procedure. There might have been some permanent cosmetic result that she didn't like. She might even be hospitalized, although this is a real rarity. These days, a serious medical problem due to a cosmetic procedure occurs for only one in several thousand patients.

135

Occasionally people even die, although this usually involves other problems, such as the alleged drug abuse implicated in the recent death of a celebrity's wife after cosmetic surgery.

As of this writing, there have been a number of deaths due to liposuction in the U.S. My feeling is that liposuction procedures should be among the safest procedures in cosmetic surgery. I feel that modern liposuction training has been lacking in some of the physicians who have experienced deaths. It is crucial to have your liposuction performed by a physician who is very familiar with the proper local anesthetic techniques. These were largely developed by dermatologists, and any doctor who performs liposuction should be familiar with dermatologic medical information.

These skin doctors developed the safest standards for liposuction surgery. In my opinion, anyone doing a modern liposuction should have heard of this, and be able to explain at least in rough terms how his or her technique is similar to or different from the dermatologists. The artful use of the tumescent fluid, which needs to be carefully spread out in all the areas to be liposuctioned, is the most critical single factor in a patient's safety. The anesthetic injection process takes in most cases over an hour to perform — that is, it takes over an hour for the tumescent fluid to be inserted underneath the skin *before* the actual liposuction procedure begins.

This is more than a matter of patient comfort; tumescent anesthetic makes possible a safer surgery and faster recovery. A patient who is only locally anesthetized can give input not possible with general anesthetic. In other words, the local anesthetic patient can often tell the doctor if something is wrong, while the completely sedated and asleep patient can't. In addition, general anesthetic causes more chance of bleeding due to the relaxation of the blood vessels of the whole body. With tumescent anesthetic, the patient bleeds less, and that helps prevent complications and promotes healing. Dermatologists often use very little sedation or relaxation medicine at all, but we give the patients a choice of sedation. Some patients choose to have no IV sedation while others prefer mild to moderate IV sedation.

Asking a doctor about his tumescent technique may be a good index of how safe his technique is overall, but there are certainly no guarantees. You must rely on your skill in judging people and use the suggestions we offer in "How to Choose a Cosmetic Surgeon" to make your decision.

Every doctor has his own profile of problems based both on the procedures he does and his overall experience. Hair transplants, for example, if done in the modern manner by the best practitioners, are very predictable. On the other hand, tummy tucks have a significantly higher problem rate no matter who does the surgery. Liposuction and fat transfer are somewhere in between. Breast implants, because a foreign substance is added to the body, have a chance of hardening and becoming unacceptable at any time during the rest of the patient's life.

Patients should understand the facts and plan for the best and the worst possibilities. Likewise, the doctor plans for his entire profile of patients, the good and the few poor results. Patients should be followed-up at no charge until they are stable and happy with the process (follow-up charges are traditionally included in the surgical fee). In my opinion, touch-ups should also be free if the patient has a significant problem.

Follow-up visits are the patient's responsibility. He or she must show up for follow-up appointments faithfully, so the doctor can spot any potential problems early.

If you can't accept the above — if you feel as though you couldn't possibly survive a long hassle with a difficult recovery — you should not have cosmetic surgery (or most elective surgeries for that matter). Chances for complications are slim, but definite.

The Hyperbaric Chamber 17

ℒ *The hyperbaric chamber is an oxygen compression tank that the patient gets in to for two hours or so every day for the first three to seven days after surgery. It can shorten surgical recovery time dramatically and help prevent complications.*

It may sound like science fiction, but we can now put patients in a specially designed oxygen compression tank that may cut healing time almost in half. It's called a hyperbaric chamber, and it's been used in medicine for over 20 years to treat a variety of problems including the decompression sickness that deep sea divers are subject to. I've been interested in its potential since the mid 1980s, when I was involved in the treatment of divers at the University of Southern California facility at Catalina Island near Los Angeles. I now use a hyperbaric chamber to improve cosmetic surgery recovery time; in fact, I was the first cosmetic surgeon in the U.S. to have one in my surgical center for use in the surgical healing process. I believe that its potential is enormous.

Here's how it works. At sea level, we live in air that bears down on our bodies at a certain weight, or pressure. You've probably noticed that when you travel to a location high in the mountains, the atmosphere changes. You may feel lightheaded or have trouble breathing, because there's actually less oxygen in the air. You're at a different *atmospheric pressure*. If you go below sea level, the pressure also changes, but instead of air pressure, it's *water* pressure. If you were under 30 feet of water, you'd have a lot of water weight pressing down on you. This is double the normal air pressure at sea level.

What the hyperbaric chamber (or tank) does is to create an atmosphere that is usually about double the pressure of normal sea level oxygen, as if you were 30 to 40 feet under water. But it's not water that's pushing down on you. It's air pressure.

To put it simply, when you're compressed to double the usual pressure using pure oxygen, the body gets "supercharged" with oxygen, and higher-than-normal amounts get into the bloodstream. This stimulates the healing process by allowing more oxygen to get delivered to the peripheral areas of the body, like the skin. Swelling decreases and new blood vessels are thought to grow faster.

Probably the most traditional use of the hyperbaric chamber has been to treat deep sea divers when they get "the bends." This happens when they've stayed down for so long that they get too much nitrogen in their blood, and when they come up, the nitrogen turns to bubbles, which causes all kinds of serious medical problems. The chamber can equalize the pressure to bring it all back to normal, and bring the diver up slowly so his body has a chance to rid itself of the nitrogen.

Victims of carbon monoxide inhalation, such as people attempting to commit suicide in a car, can sometimes be cured of their problem if a hyperbaric chamber is available. The chamber allows the person to get enough oxygen despite the carbon monoxide poisoning of the body's oxygen-carrying system.

Hyperbaric chambers are also used to treat burn victims in some hospitals. They heal skin rapidly — at perhaps almost double the usual rate. Healing from laser peels is helped in the same way. I've routinely used our hyperbaric chamber for patients who wanted a super-fast recovery so they could return to work more quickly, or look presentable for an important social engagement.

The chamber can also help other wounds heal. Doctors sometimes have to cover a hole in the skin produced by a burn, a skin cancer, or an accident. When skin is cut and brought from somewhere to cover a gap, the new area is called a "flap" or "graft." These can produce wonderful results when they heal properly, but there is always a chance that an area will die, and the wound won't close. If the patient spends enough time in the chamber — about one or two hours per day for two weeks — circulation can be increased and blood vessel growth stimulated so much that the chance of flap and graft death in most cases is nearly zero.

Professional athletes sometimes use the hyperbaric chamber by jumping into it between rounds in sports just to charge up their muscles and joints and increase their energy. Healing of athletic injuries is also improved. You may have also heard about certain celebrities who own hyperbaric chambers as well.

One avant-garde use for the chamber right now is for people who've had strokes. When a stroke occurs, a blood vessel in the brain is blocked. The chamber probably allows oxygen to go beyond the blockage, feeding those parts with much-needed oxygen. Many stroke patients who'd lost the ability to read, write, or hear, have actually become more alert and functional while in the chamber. They've been able to read or watch TV. This effect only lasts a few hours, and it's still in the experimental stages. But the belief and experience of some practitioners is that if someone has a series of treatments, perhaps 40 to 60, there can be long-term improvement. This is standard treatment in other areas of the world, such as China.

I'm a big believer in the hyperbaric chamber, which is why I'm committed to the point of actually having purchased one. I've been using it for liposuction, laser peels, fat transplant and hair transplant patients, and all heal much more quickly because of it. Bruising goes away faster, swelling decreases faster, and the patients actually feel better overall. It's exceedingly effective for laser peels. Normally it takes up to two weeks for new skin to completely grow back after a laser peel. With daily chamber treatments, this can be sometimes decreased to as little as five days. After a laser peel, lingering redness is a problem for many patients. The chamber gets rid of the red more quickly. For liposuction, the chamber helps the swelling decrease much more quickly, which results in less postoperative discomfort. We believe it also helps with fat retention after fat transplants. For hair transplants, we're hoping that the chamber will help urge the new growth through the dormant period faster, and that patients will see new hair much sooner.

Using hyperbaric medicine routinely for cosmetic surgery patients is a very new idea at this writing. One of the primary reasons is cost. Most hyperbaric centers are hospital-based, which is expensive. Outpatient centers can make the whole process more reasonable, especially when you consider that the patient gets back to work sooner.

There are other recovery aids your doctor may suggest. The Sofpulse is a large 8-inch electrical magnet which gives a comforting, mild sensation of heat when applied to an operated area for 30 minutes a day for the first few days, and it's very helpful in relieving post-procedure discomfort. The Accuscope is another useful machine which delivers a mild massage to help healing and the smoothing out of lumps. And your cosmetic surgeon should at least offer an external physical therapy ultrasound machine to help with lumpiness or swelling after the procedure.

But in addition, you should also ask about the hyper-baric chamber. I'm so impressed with its remarkable contribution to healing that I'm convinced it will become part of the cosmetic surgery mainstream very soon.

ଛ Patient Stories ℘

Ronald, age 54

I had two hair transplants and the second one, when I used the hyperbaric chamber, was very easy by comparison to the first. There was almost no swelling or pain the second time. And the hair grew right away! The doctor said that it may have just been luck or something to do with my hair, but I think it was due to the use of the chamber.

Elaine, age 34

After my second laser peel was done I stepped right into the chamber. I was healed in six days, and it took me a week and a half the first time. The redness went away more quickly, too.

What Price Beauty?

Ah, the big question. How much does all this cost? Many people scrimp and save for years to pay for cosmetic surgery, and if you're one of them, you'll want to know what to expect. I must emphasize that *prices vary widely from one doctor to the next,* and it's a huge ballpark. A doctor's fees are set according to many factors, including his overhead, his reputation, how long it takes him to perform a procedure, what the market will bear, the geographic region (a doctor in Arkansas isn't going to charge the same as a doctor in Los Angeles), the equipment he's using (it has to be able to pay for itself), how effective his marketing is, and so on.

When you shop around, remind yourself that you won't get something for nothing. If you buy the cheapest *anything,* you probably aren't satisfied. What do you own that you bought *just* on the basis of price? Most people find quality most important. After all, you are dealing with your looks, and there is a *huge* difference in quality between surgeons and procedures. Please make sure you read chapter 2 on choosing your cosmetic surgeon if you aren't convinced.

But even given all this, there is usually some room for negotiation with any surgeon. Remember that a doctor's overhead may be as much as 80 percent of his total revenue, and if he cuts his fees by 20 percent, he may not have anything left with which to feed his kids. However, if several procedures are done together, a doctor can sometimes afford to cut fees for the additional procedures by perhaps a quarter and possibly a third.

Following are some rough price ranges for 1998 surgical fees. Remember that fees vary tremendously from one doctor to the next. Facility fees may be extra — be sure to ask:

Liposuction

Look carefully at the quality you're buying, and judge mainly by the doctor's "before and after" photos. Also, your safety depends on the doctor's experience with the newest techniques (for more details, see the chapter "What's the Worst That Can Happen?"). Many doctors offer liposuction, but only a few really focus on it. If your budget is limited, you may settle for an inexperienced physician, but remember that touch-ups can be expensive, and the results often aren't as good as if it was done right originally. Price also depends on how big you are, so if you save money on groceries, you may also save on the cosmetic surgeon.

Body liposuction: $2,000 to $10,000, depending on how much of the body is treated
Chin/lower face liposuction: $1,500 to $3,500

Facial Laser Peel

An aesthetician (a manicurist or cosmetician) can do a chemical peel in a spa for as little as $50. This produces a "freshening" effect without any real wrinkle or scar relief. These procedures have a definite complication rate — and that means a chance of facial scarring — in anyone's hands. You're better off with someone who may charge a little more but knows the field better.

Full face laser peel or deep chemical peel: $2,000 to $5,000
Partial face: $750 to $1,500
Full face light Glycolic peel or light TCA peel: $200 to $500

Fat transfer

Liposuction of the donor area is usually included in the price, and sometimes a laser or chemical peel is included.

Lips alone: $500 to $1,500
Whole face: $3,500 to $15,000

Eyelid Reconstruction

Upper lids or lower lids alone: $1,500 to $2,500
All four lids: $2,000 to $5,000

Face Lift

$1,000 to $25,000 (I'd recommend avoiding the $1,000 surgeon)
Most are between $5,000 to $6,000

Nose job

$3,500 to $8,000 is usual. Sometimes insurance can pay a portion if your breathing is impaired

Chin Augmentation/Reduction

Alloplastic chin implant: about $1,500
Genioplasty: $2,500 to $10,000

Hair Transplant

Most patients receive about 1,200 to 1,500 grafts per session, and need 2,000 to 3,000 ultimately.

Per graft: $4 to $60

Breast Implants

This is expensive because of silicone litigation. The implant itself represents about five dollars worth of plastic, but its cost to the doctor is about $1,500.

Cost to the patient: $4,500 to $7,500

Veins

Some doctors claim that they can eliminate most of the veins in one session.

Injections: $200 to $1,000 per session
Larger veins: $1,500 to $2,500 per leg

Hyperbaric Treatments

Three to five treatments are needed for routine healing after a procedure. Each session is usually at 2 or 2.4 "atmospheres" at 100 percent oxygen, and lasts one to two hours. Price shop for this one.

Per treatment: $200 to $1,000

Other Laser Treatments

There are various prices, and generally several sessions are needed to treat a particular problem.

Per session: $400 to $1,000

Cellulite Therapy

Just like a good massage, with 20 to 40 sessions needed.

Per session: $50 to $100

The Brave New World of Anti-Aging Drugs and Diets

   The new anti-aging medicines and diets may be even more effective than cosmetic surgery for people who want to look and feel younger.

   Human Growth Hormone (HGH) is lower in people over 40, and some doctors are now prescribing "replacement" HGH, just as the female hormones are replaced by synthetic estrogen after menopause. Remarkable improvement in the patients' sense of well-being and in muscle and organ functioning may occur. The long-term effects are unknown. Some doctors are convinced it will lengthen the life span.

   Consult your physician for advice about these drugs. This information is changing all the time, and the safety of these medications hasn't been completely established. This chapter is just a preview of a complex field and shouldn't be used for medical advice. I'm very optimistic, however, that many of these medications will assume a major role in medicine in the near future.

Cosmetic surgery is all about looking and feeling better, and often about looking and feeling *younger*. While the surgeons have been working on their new techniques, the medical doctors haven't been asleep. Here's the story about the new life-enhancement and prolongation medicines that may quickly become a routine part of your medical and surgical care. It sounds like science fiction, but a lot of this may soon transform people even more than surgery.

The most exciting news is Human Growth Hormone (HGH). This medication was formerly used to stimulate growth in children who grew too slowly. Until recently, it was not approved by our conservative Food and Drug Administration for other conditions. It was well known to professional body-builders, however, for muscle enhancement, but unlike steroids, it's "natural" and can't be detected currently with blood testing.

After a person is about 40 years old, the amount of HGH in the body declines dramatically, and many of the effects of aging seem to be caused by this decline in HGH. Some doctors have been using this drug for "replacement" in these normal aging people. A few cosmetic surgeons are also using it during the few weeks following surgery to speed healing.

My "take" on the medical literature is that this hormone is helpful for many problems. Also, the patients' stories are remarkable. It has been claimed to restore vigor, sexuality, energy, muscles, and also to slowly get rid of fat without a change in diet or exercise patterns. All the organs of the body may grow a little in size, reversing the trend that comes with aging, and it is also a therapy for osteoporosis (thinning of the bone structure). There are even rumors that it helps reverse or stabilize cataracts. There are very few known side effects with it after decades of experience using it on children, and several years experience with older people. It's now manufactured to be exactly like the HGH the body pro-duces. Unfortunately, it has to be given, like insulin, in injection form, and currently costs up to $200 a week. Prices should come down very soon.

We have to be careful about early judgments, however. Every physician has seen drugs touted early on as the cure for everything up to and including hangovers, which later proved to have some big problem. But the early studies and stories about HGH are very encouraging. I have a 55-year-old physician friend who has been using it for six months and he says that he's lost 20 pounds and feels great. He says his sexuality is "crazy like a 16-year-old's." People over 40 should watch developments in this area carefully. I think we may be headed for major breakthroughs with HGH, both in longevity and the quality of life.

Even if you don't have $8,000 per year to shell out for HGH, you might try melatonin. It's an over-the-counter pill, and very cheap. This hormone may be the master sleep regulator. The amount of melatonin in the body falls dramatically between 30 and 40 years old, and it is given as replacement therapy by some physicians specializing in anti-aging. It seems to really help sleep, and has been used widely to treat jet lag (taken at 8 p.m. in the time zone you're entering). Effective doses are many times the three milligram tablet that is available. Consult your doctor for advice.

"Anti-oxidant" vitamins are thought by some to "scavenge free radicals" or clean up molecular destruction in the body. I think the evidence for this is not as strong as most of the topics in this chapter, but there doesn't seem to be any harm in taking vitamins if the doses are not too high. Make your own judgments; this can get expensive and I don't have a final opinion now. I do, however, take vitamins myself.

DHEA is a hormone that is the starting point for the biological manufacture of many of the hormones that regulate your body's function. Because hormones in the body decrease with age, physicians are now supplementing their patients' diets with DHEA. It is taken orally, it's inexpensive, and it seems to have a positive effect on overall functioning and energy levels.

The female hormones estrogen and progesterone have been used routinely for over a decade for supplementation of women past menopause or "change of life," or after a complete hysterectomy which removed the ovaries. Although this is standard medical care, only about 10 to 20 percent of women who should be supplemented are actually taking their pills or using the newer "patch" that supplies the drug through the skin. This is unfortunate, because the medicines have many helpful effects including partial protection from osteoporosis and heart disease. Although estrogen alone can increase the risk of uterine cancer, when used in combination with progesterone the overall risk actually drops. Some studies showed a very small increase in breast cancer rates, but these have been outweighed by many studies which show no effect. If you have breast cancer already, however, no female hormone supplementation is generally recommended.

Testosterone is, of course, the male sexual hormone, made mainly in the testicles. Now, a new testosterone gel or patch is used on the surface of the skin, so shots are no longer needed to treat testosterone deficiency. Some doctors think that this hormone helps prevent osteoporosis and heart disease as well as aiding sexuality and having many other effects. There is a blood test to see how much the body has left, and if levels are low, some longevity doctors will use supplementation. Some specialists use it often for men over 40.

The fear with some of these medicines is that their use will shut off production of normal hormones by the body. Doctors usually give "drug holidays" to patients — periods in which no medicine is taken —in order to let the body recover and produce natural hormones.

What about the new diets? Although from the hype they look like fads, high protein diets seem to be based on science. Popularized in *Entering the Zone* and *Mastering the Zone* by Barry Sears and *Protein Power* by Michael and Mary Eades, the new balanced carbohydrate-fat-protein diets claim to regulate the production of two key body hormones, glucagon and insulin. These diets recommend more fat and protein and less carbohydrate than either the standard recommended high carbohydrate diet, the American Heart Association diet, or the American Diabetic Association diet.

We also like *Maximum Metabolism,* by Robert M. Giller, M.D. He goes into some detail about eating carbohydrates in the morning instead of the evening and how caffeine stimulates insulin (the "hunger hormone"). He points out that besides burning calories, exercise stabilizes insulin and blood sugar. It also stimulates the production of hormones that make you feel fuller by raising the blood fat level. As your muscle mass increases, you can eat more without gaining fat. His psychological suggestions for weight loss are excellent.

The idea is that human beings aren't naturally grain eaters and that high protein sources such as animal proteins are generally healthier. When we stay away from dense carbohydrates like bread, we are less hungry and tend to lose weight naturally given a balanced fat consumption. This has been known for years. You may remember that the Atkins diet was based on the natural lack of hunger that occurs when people eat more protein and cut down on carbohydrates. I think the science for these diets is pretty respectable, and I've been recommending them to my patients. Many competitive athletes also find these diets useful.

As much as I hate to say this, all of these medical advances may soon overshadow cosmetic surgery for their anti-aging effects. They're not going to change the shape of your nose, or give you big breasts, but in the over 40 age group, a year of HGH might have more of an effect on your shape than liposuction.

New Developments in Liposuction 20

🔖 *Ultrasonic liposuction is new, but is it better? From what we've seen, probably not.*

🔖 *New lipo tool design is making procedures faster and thus probably safer. But the surgeon's technique is more important than any other factor.*

🔖 *Madeline's disease, a condition where multiple balls of fat grow all over the body, can also be treated with liposuction.*

The New Ultrasonic Liposuction — Is it an Improvement?

Since 1996, ultrasonic liposuction has been widely advertised. There are two types: internal and external ultrasonic liposuction. With internal ultrasonic liposuction, a cannula that is specially designed to transmit ultrasound waves is inserted into a person's fat and moved around, and the fat is broken up. Large holes need to be placed in the skin to use the large ultrasonic liposuction instrument. This machine costs around $40,000 and makes the procedure somewhat easier for the physician. The physician does not have to use all the muscle power to push the cannula past resistance. Instead, the cannula glides into the tissues.

External ultrasonic liposuction involves using a machine such as a chiropractor or physical therapist might use. A probe is placed on the surface of the skin. This probe helps somewhat to break up the fat. This may make the cannulas go into the fat a little more easily, and some physicians have reported improved skin results in a shorter time interval. Generally, our understanding of external ultrasonic liposuction is that it is a minimal improvement, and our experience with liposuction using this treatment has been unimpressive. Obviously, the amount of energy delivered through the skin has to be a small amount because the ultrasound machines can burn the skin surface if too much energy is used.

The medical journals have published many reports of problems patients have after internal ultrasonic liposuction. It appears that sometimes complications occur in as many as 50 percent of patients who have this procedure. These problems, such as seromas (fluid collections underneath the skin) and prolonged time off work due to pain, are not generally life threatening but can be quite irritating. In addition, many physicians have reported skin burns. A great number of physicians who were initially enthusiastic about this have given it up. Lots of experience is necessary to safely use internal ultrasonic liposuction. Also, many of the benefits that were initially thought to occur due to the ultrasound seem to be actually as a result of using the tumescent anesthetic. As you know, the most sophisticated surgeons have been using tumescent anesthetic for five to ten years, but there have been many surgeons who have not learned this technique until ultrasonic liposuction appeared.

My feeling about this technology is that it is probably not an improvement. Our small cannula liposuction is still superior. In the *American Journal of Cosmetic Surgery*, Volume 14, Number 3 (1997), Dr. Gerard Boutboul remarked,

. . . Ultrasound is being pushed by influential commercial advertising supported by very few clinical experiences showing no proof of the superiority of the ultrasound. . . . As I reported during the American Academy of Cosmetic Surgery Congress in Palm Springs . . . ultrasonic lipoplasty is about to disappear. . . . [A]fter treating more than 300 cases, we have stopped using this technique because of the many problems and no evidence of clinical superiority over a classic lipoplasty.

Once again, I wish to tell American doctors using the ultrasound technique to be aware of its dangers as well as an absence of progress when compared to simple lipoplasty using micro cannulas, tumescent technique, and crossed planes.

Also, the *European Academy of Cosmetic Surgery Newsletter* (winter 1997) reported

The ultrasound liposuction which is mostly abandoned here in Europe because of its unsatisfactory results and high burns is now trying to sell in America. As the European Academy of Cosmetic Surgery, we want to continue to declare the traditional liposuction with small cannulas and the super wet technique as the most safe, effective, and affordable technique of body contouring until a scientific study proves that another technique is to be superior to the traditional liposuction.

An Unusual Case for Liposuction

At the end of the photo section is an example of the versatility of modern liposuction. The man pictured has an unusual condition called "lipomatosis," or Madeline's disease, a condition where multiple balls of fat grow all over a person's body. These balls of fat continue to grow throughout the patient's lifetime. Treatment in the past has been to cut large holes in the skin and cut out the fat balls. These growths range from the size of small marbles to the size of grapefruits. Medical treatment has been used, but is only partially successful. A medicine called Albuterol,® taken in pill form, helps slow the growth of these noncancerous tumors and sometimes stops them all together. This patient was treated with standard liposuction techniques and did very well.

The Cosmetic Surgery Junkie

"Doctor, what else do I need?"

This is a frequently asked question after a patient has had a satisfactory result from a procedure. The correct answer often is: more may be a mistake. Most of us have just a few areas that can be significantly improved through cosmetic surgery. Very few patients would benefit from every possible procedure. Often after a positive experience and a great result, patients become more trusting of the surgeon and also more critical of their bodies' flaws. They will frequently seek surgeries that are not always as appropriate as the first, and must be cautioned against becoming addicted to the process.

Because this is elective or voluntary surgery, the patient is responsible to a large extent for what gets done. But the doctor should refuse inappropriate requests and counsel about potential problems. You must bear in mind two other factors when you're dealing with doctors. First, most surgeons love to do surgery of any kind. Second, although most doctors try to put the patient first, they have financial pressures. And patients are very trusting. So if the doctor leaves you with any negative feelings about your procedure, you should listen carefully. He's doing his job and he has your best interests at heart.

One of our patients in her late thirties came in for one surgery and had an excellent result. She went to consult with someone for rhinoplasty (which we don't do) and ended up with cheek implants, chin implant, rhinoplasty, and face lift all at once. (These are done routinely together and can be appropriate for some patients.) She developed scarring and a strange appearance and came back to me hoping that I could somehow take her back to the way she was before she had the surgeries. She was disappointed to find that unfortunately I couldn't help her.

"Touch-up" procedures of almost any kind are more difficult and less likely to produce a happy result. Secondary face lifts, rhinoplasty, and liposuction all have a higher chance of complications and are not as predictable, even with a skilled doctor. It's safer to go to the best and thus make a correction procedure unlikely. Some physicians, for example, do secondary surgeries after 25 percent of their own liposuction cases! (Some surgeons even tell their lipo patients that they will need several touch-ups to attain their goal. A reasonable lipo touch-up rate is one in 20.) And, if you gain weight after your lipo, don't think that it will be easy to remove it again. It doesn't work that way. Sometimes we can help, but not always. The areas already worked on are tougher and often don't respond as well. You must do your best to take care of yourself properly and stay fit. Try not to get into the "multiple touch-up syndrome" after any surgery. You may gradually look worse.

If you go to several doctors — a good thing sometimes — carefully evaluate each one according to our instructions and don't immediately trust the new physician because you've had a great experience with the last. Make your best judgements about what you need in light of all the information you can gather, including what the physician says. If you hear from reputable sources that you're not a candidate for a procedure, try to accept that. Don't look around for someone else to do the surgery.

When you go out to a nice restaurant, you don't eat everything on the menu. By the same token, at the doctor's office, you don't need to have every cosmetic surgery under the sun. You'll do better if you control yourself and exercise some common sense. Be careful out there.

Index

For more information, contact

ROBERT A. YOHO, M.D.

Voice: (626) 585-0800
Fax: (626) 585-8887
Website: http://www.DrYoho.com/

675 S. Arroyo Parkway, Suite 100
Pasadena, California 91105